MONOGRAPHS ON POPULATION AGING

General Editors
Bernard Jeune and James W. Vaupel

Vol. 1
*Development of Oldest-Old Mortality, 1950-1990:*
*Evidence from 28 Developed Countries*
Väinö Kannisto

Vol. 2
*Exceptional Longevity:*
*From Prehistory to the Present*
Bernard Jeune and James W. Vaupel (editors)

Vol. 3
*The Advancing Frontier of Survival:*
*Life Tables for Old Age*
Väinö Kannisto

Vol. 4
*Population Data at a Glance:*
*Shaded Contour Maps of Demographic Surfaces over Age and Time*
James W. Vaupel, Wang Zhenglian, Kirill F. Andreev,
and Anatoli I. Yashin

*Aging Research Center*
*Centre for Health and Social Policy*
*Odense University*

# Population Data at a Glance:
Shaded Contour Maps of Demographic Surfaces over Age and Time

*James W. Vaupel, Wang Zhenglian, Kirill F. Andreev, and Anatoli I. Yashin*

*Odense Monographs on Population Aging, 4.*
Odense University Press

*Population Data at a Glance:*
*Shaded Contour Maps of Demographic Surfaces over Age and Time*
James W. Vaupel, Wang Zhenglian, Kirill F. Andreev, and Anatoli I. Yashin
Printed by Special-Trykkeriet Viborg a-s, Denmark
Cover illustration: Adam and Eve (with whom the demography of birth, death, and migration began) by Sonia Brandes
Layout by Susanne Kløjgaard
ISBN 87-7838-338-2
ISSN 0909-119X

Odense University Press
Campusvej 55
DK-5230 Odense M
Phone +45 66 15 79 99 Fax +45 66 15 81 26
E-mail: Press@forlag.ou.dk

# Contents

List of figures . . . . . . . . . . . . . . . . . . . . . . . . . . . . . . . . . . . . . . . . . . . . . 6
Preface . . . . . . . . . . . . . . . . . . . . . . . . . . . . . . . . . . . . . . . . . . . . . . . . . 17
Acknowledgements . . . . . . . . . . . . . . . . . . . . . . . . . . . . . . . . . . . . . . 18

    1. Introduction . . . . . . . . . . . . . . . . . . . . . . . . . . . . . . . . . . . . . . . 19
    2. The evolution of Italian male mortality . . . . . . . . . . . . . . . . . . . . . . 21
    3. Levels, shades, and grids . . . . . . . . . . . . . . . . . . . . . . . . . . . . . . 24
    4. Smoothed maps . . . . . . . . . . . . . . . . . . . . . . . . . . . . . . . . . . . . 27
    5. Close-ups . . . . . . . . . . . . . . . . . . . . . . . . . . . . . . . . . . . . . . . . 31
    6. Maps from interpolated data . . . . . . . . . . . . . . . . . . . . . . . . . . . . 35
    7. Maps of female fertility . . . . . . . . . . . . . . . . . . . . . . . . . . . . . . . 40
    8. Alternative graphic displays of US female fertility . . . . . . . . . . . . . . 47
    9. The female populations of Sweden and Japan at older ages . . . . . . . . . 49
   10. Relative surfaces of Italian mortality, US fertility,
        and Belgian population . . . . . . . . . . . . . . . . . . . . . . . . . . . . . . . 52
   11. Small multiples . . . . . . . . . . . . . . . . . . . . . . . . . . . . . . . . . . . . 57
   12. Ratio surfaces . . . . . . . . . . . . . . . . . . . . . . . . . . . . . . . . . . . . . 65
   13. Sex ratios, nuptiality, and cause-specific mortality . . . . . . . . . . . . . . 68
   14. Life table statistics for Belgian females . . . . . . . . . . . . . . . . . . . . . 73
   15. US female mortality rates from 1900 to 2050 . . . . . . . . . . . . . . . . . . 77
   16. Oldest-old mortality . . . . . . . . . . . . . . . . . . . . . . . . . . . . . . . . . 77
   17. Checking data quality . . . . . . . . . . . . . . . . . . . . . . . . . . . . . . . . 85
   18. High Danish mortality . . . . . . . . . . . . . . . . . . . . . . . . . . . . . . . 89
   19. Conclusion . . . . . . . . . . . . . . . . . . . . . . . . . . . . . . . . . . . . . . . 94

References . . . . . . . . . . . . . . . . . . . . . . . . . . . . . . . . . . . . . . . . . . . . 96

# List of figures

Figure 1. Probabilities of death for Italian males,
from age 0 to 99 and year 1886 to 1986
- a. In color . . . . . . . . . . . . . . . . . . . . . . . . . . . . . . . . . . . . . . . . . . . . 22
- b. As *Figure 1(a)*, but in black and white . . . . . . . . . . . . . . . . . . . . . . . . . 23
- c. As *Figure 1(b)*, but with 10 contour lines . . . . . . . . . . . . . . . . . . . . . . . 25
- d. As *Figure 1(b)*, but with evenly spaced contour lines . . . . . . . . . . . . . . . . 26
- e. As *Figure 1(b)*, but with 17 contour lines . . . . . . . . . . . . . . . . . . . . . . . 26
- f. As *Figure 1(b)*, but with a grid . . . . . . . . . . . . . . . . . . . . . . . . . . . . . 28
- g. As *Figure 1(b)*, but without contour lines . . . . . . . . . . . . . . . . . . . . . . . 29
- h. As *Figure 1(b)*, but without shading . . . . . . . . . . . . . . . . . . . . . . . . . . 29
- i. As *Figure 1(b)*, but smoothed on a 5 x 5 square . . . . . . . . . . . . . . . . . . . 32
- j. As *Figure 1(b)*, but smoothed on a 11 x 11 square . . . . . . . . . . . . . . . . . 33
- k. As *Figure 1(b)*, but smoothed on a weighted 5 x 5 square . . . . . . . . . . . . 33
- l. As *Figure 1(b)*, but with only three contour lines . . . . . . . . . . . . . . . . . . 34

Figure 2. Probabilities of death for Italian males
- a. With a grid, from age 10 to 49 and year 1910 to 1969 . . . . . . . . . . . . . . . 36
- b. As *Figure 2(a)*, but with different contour lines . . . . . . . . . . . . . . . . . . . 36
- c. For cohorts, from age 0 to 54 and year of birth 1894 to 1924 . . . . . . . . . . 37
- d. As *Figure 2(c)*, but relative to 1903 cohort age-specific levels,
  from age 0 to 54 and year of birth 1904 to 1909 . . . . . . . . . . . . . . . . . . . 37

Figure 3. Probabilities of death for Italian males,
from age 0 to 79 and year 1881 to 1964 . . . . . . . . . . . . . 38
- a. Interpolated data
- b. Single-year-of-time-and-age data

Figure 4. Probabilities of death for Swedish females,
   from age 0 to 79 and year 1778 to 1993 .............. 39

Figure 5. US birth rates, from age 14 to 49
   and year 1917 to 1990 .......................... 41

Figure 6. US cohort birth rates, from age 14 to 49
   and year of birth 1867 to 1977 ................... 42

Figure 7. US birth rates by current year and year
   of birth, from current year 1917 to 1990
   and year of birth 1867 to 1977 ................... 43

Figure 8. Chinese birth rates, from age 15 to 49
   and year 1940 to 1989 .......................... 44

Figure 9. Finnish birth rates, from age 15 to 49
   and year 1776 to 1970 .......................... 45

Figure 10. Alternative graphic displays of US birth rates .... 46
    a. US birth rates from year 1917 to 1990 at ages 18, 23, and 28
    b. US birth rates from age 14 to 49 in years 1920, 1950, and 1980
    c. Three-dimensional perspective for ages 14 to 49 and years 1917 to 1990

Figure 11. Three-dimensional plots of US birth rates ....... 48

Figure 12. Swedish female population from year 1861 to 1993
    a. Population from age 0 to 111 ................................. 49
    b. Population relative to average level in 1861-1870,
       from age 0 to 100 .......................................... 50

Figure 13. Japanese female population from age 80 to 116
    and year 1950 to 1991 ........................... 51

Figure 14. Probabilities of death for Italian males
    relative to age-specific 1925 levels,
    from age 0 to 99 and year 1886 to 1986 .............. 52

Figure 15. US birth rates relative to age-specific 1980 levels,
    from age 14 to 45 and year 1917 to 1990 ............. 53

Figure 16. Probabilities of death for Italian males
relative to infant mortality levels,
from age 0 to 99 and year 1886 to 1986 .............. 54

Figure 17. Age-distribution of Belgian female population,
from age 0 to 99 and year 1892 to 1977 .............. 55

Figure 18. Cumulative distribution of US births by age
and year, from age 14 to 49 and year 1917 to 1990 ..... 56

Figure 19. Cumulative distribution of US births by age
and year of birth of mother, from age 14 to 49
and year of birth 1903 to 1940 ..................... 56

Figure 20. US parity-specific birth rates,
from age 14 to 49 and year 1917 to 1980 ............. 58
    a. At parity 1
    b. At parity 2
    c. At parity 3
    d. At parity 4
    e. At parity 5
    f. At parity 6

Figure 21. Probabilities of death for males and females
in Italy, Belgium, and France, from age 15 to age 49
and year 1910 to 1965 .......................... 60
   a. Italian male
   b. Italian female
   c. Belgian male
   d. Belgian female
   e. French male
   f. French female

Figure 22. Probabilities of death relative to 1870
age-specific levels, for males and females in Italy,
Sweden, and England and Wales, from age 5 to 79
and year 1870 to 1978 .......................... 61
   a. Italian male
   b. Italian female
   c. Swedish male
   d. Swedish female
   e. English and Welsh male
   f. English and Welsh female

Figure 23. Probabilities of death in Sweden relative to age-
specific levels from 1778 to 1799, from age 0 to 79
and year 1778 to 1993 .......................... 62
   a. Male
   b. Female

Figure 24. Probabilities of death relative to 1870 age-specific cohort levels, for males and females in Italy, Sweden, and England and Wales, from age 5 to 79 and year 1870 to 1978 ........................... 64
    a. Italian male
    b. Italian female
    c. Swedish male
    d. Swedish female
    e. English and Welsh male
    f. English and Welsh female

Figure 25. Probabilities of death for Italian females divided by Italian male probabilities, from age 0 to 99 and year 1886 to 1986 .............. 66
    a. With contour lines at multiples of 1.1 from 0.513 to 1.21
    b. With selected contour lines from 0.909 to 1.1

Figure 26. Probabilities of death for French males divided by probabilities for Italian males ............. 67
    a. From age 10 to 70 and year 1900 to 1960
    b. As *Figure 26(a)*, but smoothed on a weighted 5 x 5 square

Figure 27. US birth rates at parity 1 minus those at parity 2, from age 14 to 49 and year 1917 to 1980 ...... 68

Figure 28. Belgian female population divided by
   Belgian male population, from age 0 to 99
   and year 1892 to 1977 ............................ 69

Figure 29. Chinese female first marriage rates,
   from age 15 to 35 ............................. 70
   a. From year 1950 to 1987
   b. Smoothed and conditional, from year 1970 to 1987

Figure 30. Death rates from tuberculosis for males
   in England and Wales, from age 0 to 79
   and year 1861 to 1964 ............................ 71

Figure 31. Belgian female population, from age 0 to 99
   and year 1892 to 1977 ............................ 72

Figure 32. Belgian female deaths, from age 0 to 99
   and year 1892 to 1977 ............................ 74

Figure 33. Probabilities of death for Belgian females,
   from age 0 to 99 and year 1892 to 1977 .............. 74

Figure 34. Belgian female period survivorship,
from age 0 to 99 and year 1892 to 1977 .............. 75

Figure 35. Belgian female period life expectancy,
from age 0 to 99 and year 1892 to 1977 .............. 75

Figure 36. Belgian female cohort survivorship,
from age 0 to 99 and year 1892 to 1977 .............. 76
   a. By current year and age
   b. By year of birth and age

Figure 37. Force of mortality for US males and females
based on Faber (1982) life tables, from age 0 to 84
and year 1900 to 2080 ......................... 78
   a. Males
   b. Females

Figure 38. Force of mortality of US males and females
relative to 1980 age-specific levels, from age 0 to 84
and year 1900 to 2080 ......................... 79
   a. Males
   b. Females

Figure 39. Force of mortality in Sweden,
from year 1861 to 1991 .......................... 81
- a. Female, from age 80 to 111
- b. Male, from age 80 to 108

Figure 40. Force of mortality in England and Wales,
from year 1911 to 1991 .......................... 82
- a. Female, from age 80 to 114
- b. Male, from age 80 to 112

Figure 41. Force of mortality in Japan,
from year 1950 to 1991 .......................... 83
- a. Female, from age 80 to 116
- b. Male, from age 80 to 110

Figure 42. Force of mortality in aggregate of 13
countries, from year 1950 to 1990 .................. 84
- a. Female, from age 80 to 116
- b. Male, from age 80 to 112

Figure 43. Data quality checks for Spanish males,
from age 80 to 108 and year 1950 to 1986 ............. 86
- a. Period comparison with adjacent years
- b. Period comparison with adjacent ages

Figure 44. Data quality checks for Swedish males,
from age 50 to 107 and year 1861 to 1991 ............ 88
    a. Period comparison with adjacent years
    b. Period comparison with adjacent ages


Figure 45. Ratio of central death rates in Denmark
to those in Norway, from age 0 to 99 and year
1870 to 1992
    a. Males ................................................. 90
    b. Females ............................................... 91


Figure 46. Ratio of central death rates in Denmark
to those in Japan, from age 0 to 99 and year
1951 to 1990
    a. Males ................................................. 92
    b. Females ............................................... 93

# Preface

At one time, the limits of demographic research were set by the data available. Some results could be obtained by analysis of birth and death registrations and censuses, but only for the few countries for which these were available and for the few breakdowns that were permitted by the tabulating equipment in existence. With so little data available, analysis by hand methods was perfectly feasible.

Now, there are masses of data, so the problem has shifted: the due consideration and interpretation of data is a major difficulty. Under the guidance of James Vaupel and Anatoli Yashin, methods have been developed that provide interpretation at a glance. In respect of Sweden, for instance, mortality data are available for some 80 ages for more than two centuries. To look at 17 000 numbers and draw out their meaning is a major research enterprise in itself. Yet, with the methods used in this monograph all that information is contained in a single contour map.

The method has antecedents that go all the way back to Descartes' insight that mathematical functions are represented on a plane. From that it is only a step to showing empirical curves on a plane, and then go on to three dimensions, as these contour maps do. Stages in this progression were diagrams by Perozzo and Lexis that show a population as lines on the age-time plane. Arthur and Vaupel (1984), building on Preston and Coale (1982), generalized the Lexis diagram to a Lexis surface.

The material that follows makes ingenious use of computation and takes advantage of many antecedent forms of diagrams. It is presented in this monograph neither for its originality as a method, nor for the exhibition of programming skill. The drawings here appeal by reason of their substantive interest. Whether mortality improvement takes place by cohorts or by periods; at what historical periods has the fall in mortality been most striking; was the baby boom after World War II due to more births to women in the prime ages, say the 20s, or was it due to longer continuance of childbearing by women in their 30s? These and many other issues are raised in the text, but that text is suggestive rather than exhaustive, and the maps can well be used as a basis for further research.

Nathan Keyfitz

# Acknowledgements

Much of the research presented in this monograph was conducted at the International Institute for Applied Systems Analysis (IIASA) in Austria as part of a project directed by James W. Vaupel and Anatoli I. Yashin. The text is similar to the text, written by James W. Vaupel, of a IIASA research report (RR-87-16) published in July 1987. The text has been somewhat updated, some material has been deleted and some new sections have been added. By and large, however, the text has been left much the same as it was a decade ago, as has the Preface by Nathan Keyfitz.

The maps presented in the IIASA report were produced by a computer program that was developed by Bradley A. Gambill under Vaupel's supervision at Duke University and at IIASA. The maps presented here were produced by a new computer program, LEXISMAP, that was developed by Wang Zhenglian at Odense University.

Kirill Andreev, also at Odense University, developed the next version of this software. Using it, he produced a diskette for Windows that contains all the maps presented in this monograph plus some additional maps. The diskette is included with this monograph. All the maps plus further maps can also be accessed at the world-wide-web site www.demogr.mpg.de of the Max Planck Institute for Demographic Research. These new maps are superior to the printed maps in this monograph. They are large and in color. The colors and the contour lines can be changed. Interesting regions of age and time can be magnified. New datasets, e.g. for Sweden and Denmark, provide clearer, cleaner information. It is apparent that the approach, only a decade old, taken to produce the maps printed in this monograph, is obsolete. Nonetheless, printed books with black-and-white illustrations are still of substantial value and this monograph, dated as it is, is of interest, both in itself and as a supplement to the enclosed diskette.

Four research assistants at IIASA, Alan J. Bernstein, Ann E. Gowan, Mark Harris, and John M. Owen helped prepare the data bases and made useful suggestions. Jens Lauritsen, Axel Skytthe, Ivan Iachine and Zeng Xu Hui at Odense University made similar contributions, and Bernard Jeune helped supervise publication. We thank Nathan Keyfitz, Graziella Caselli, W. Brian Arthur, Dianne Goodwin, Gustav Feichtinger, Jan Hoem, Wolfgang Lutz, Gun Stenflo, Michael A. Stoto, Waldo Tobler, Jacques Vallin, Andrew Foster, Nedka Gateva, Arno Kitts, Eva Lelievre, Lucky Tedrow, John Wilmoth, and Zeng Yi for comments, Susan Stock and Kirsten M. Gauthier for secretarial assistance, Susanne Kløjgaard for help with layout and graphic design, and Sonia Brandes for the cover illustration of Adam and Eve.

# 1. Introduction

Shaded contour maps, which are widely used to depict spatial patterns, can be readily adapted to represent any surface that is defined over two dimensions. In particular, an array of demographic data can often be pictured in an intelligible and graphically striking way by a shaded contour map. The data might pertain to population levels or to rates of fertility, marriage, divorce, migration, morbidity, or mortality. Most often the data are structured by age and time - e.g., age-specific death rates over time - but in some cases other dimensions might be used, such as life expectancy or population growth rate.

Shaded contour maps permit visualization of population surfaces and offer a panoramic view impossible to obtain from the usual graphs of levels or rates at selected ages over time or at selected times over age. Furthermore, a contour map is often superior to a three-dimensional perspective plot in providing a clear, yet rich, representation of a demographic surface; it is usually difficult on a three-dimensional plot to discern the exact position of the surface above the age and time dimensions; also three-dimensional plots become confusing if made too detailed. Contour maps are particularly effective in highlighting patterns in the interaction of age, period, and cohort effects.

Shaded contour maps have been used only occasionally by demographers, in part because of the computational effort required, in part because of the lack of detailed data over long stretches of age and time, and in part because the advantages of working with population surfaces have not been fully appreciated. The use of shaded contour maps (without contour lines) is implicit in some of Lexis' (1875, 1880) original diagrams, as discussed by Dupaquier and Dupaquier (1985). In their influential study of changes in death rates over time, Kermack et al. (1934) superimpose on three of their tables some rough lines that are, in effect, contours of relative mortality. The pioneering study by Delaporte (1941) includes a set of contour maps that summarize mortality patterns in several European countries; Federici (1955) directs attention to Delaporte's contour maps in her survey of demographic methods.

Three developments should lead to greater use of demographic contour maps in the future. First, advances in computers, including the proliferation of inexpensive microcomputers and high-quality printers, are providing demographers with convenient computational power and graphical capababilities. Second, extensive arrays of population statistics are being collected, published, and put on computer diskettes and other storage devices; some of these data are by single year of age and time [e.g., Natale and Bernassola (1973), Vallin (1973), Heuser (1976, 1984), Veys (1983), and Kannisto (1994)]. Finally, there is growing recognition among demographers of the usefulness of population surfaces. Demographers have drawn three-dimensional representations of population densities at least since Berg (1860), Perozzo (1880), and Lotka (1926, 1931): more recently, an article by Arthur and Vaupel (1984), building on important research by Bennett and Horiuchi (1981) and Preston and Coale (1982), focused attention on the conceptual and analytical advantages of population surfaces.

Arthur and Vaupel (1984) introduced the phrase "Lexis surface" to describe a surface of demographic rates defined over age and time and we continue that usage here. Specific kinds of surfaces are called mortality surfaces, fertility surfaces, and so on, as appropriate, and we use interchangeably the equivalent phrases Lexis surface, population surface, and demographic surface as generic terms to describe any kind of surface pertaining to some population parameter. Because of this usage of Lexis surface and because, as noted above, the use of shaded contour maps of population surfaces is implicit in some of Lexis' diagrams, we use Lexis map as a synonym for shaded contour map.

This monograph presents a bouquet of Lexis maps to suggest the broad potential of their use in population studies. The value of such maps lies in their substantive import. They provide demographers with visual access to data that shed light on significant patterns and trends in population levels, death rates, birth rates, and other demographic parameters. In the following text, we point to some of the more interesting substantive features of the maps, to suggest the worth of such maps in population studies.

Every picture presented deserves a thousand words or more of explanation and analysis and we hope that demographers will exploit the maps as a rich lode for research. Several steps in this direction have already been taken. Caselli et al. (1985a) analyzed Lexis maps of Italian mortality and Zeng Yi et al. (1985, 1994) analyzed Lexis maps of Chinese marriage and fertility rates. At IIASA Gateva used Lexis maps to depict evolving trends in age-specific population levels in different regions of Bulgaria and Tremblay applied the maps in a study of linguistic mobility in Canada. In Wilmoth's (1985) study of age, period, and cohort effects in Italian female mortality, Lexis maps of various kinds of changes and residuals are intriguingly suggestive and revealing. Caselli et al. (1985b) compare patterns of French versus Italian mortality by using Lexis maps. Finally, to mention just one more example, Yashin used contour maps to analyze twin mortality: the lifespan of one twin is on one axis and the lifespan of the second is on the other.

As a compilation of data, the demographic maps displayed in this research monograph might be compared with the demographic tables presented in Keyfitz and Flieger (1968, 1990) or Preston et al. (1972), and we hope that the maps will prove to be useful complements to such tabular compendiums. The typical map in this monograph is based on more than 6000 data points, and some of the maps summarize considerably more data: Figure 4 is based on 17,000 points and the small multiples in Figure 22 present close to 40,000 data values. Some 100 maps are included in this monograph, so that the maps collectively display roughly 600,000 values. Each page of tables in Keyfitz and Flieger (1968) contains about 625 statistics and there are about 650 pages of tables, amounting to roughly 400,000 values. Similarly, each page of tables in Preston et al. (1972) contains about 575 statistics, on average, and there are more than 700 tables, for a grand total, once again, of roughly 400,000 values.

## 2. The evolution of Italian male mortality

Figure 1 displays the contours of mortality for Italian males from age 0 to 99 and for years 1886-1986. The Lexis map is based on probabilities of death, $q$, for single years of age and time that were calculated from cohort data assembled by Natale and Bernassola (1973) and Caselli et al. (1985a). These measures of mortality are equal to the proportion of persons born in a particular calendar year and alive at exact age $x$ who died before their $x + 1$-st birthday. This type of probability refers to events that affect each single-year cohort at each age in two successive calendar years; for a discussion of this, see Vallin (1973) or Wunsch and Termote (1978). The map, in the space of half a page or so, summarizes 100 x 100, or some ten thousand, probabilities of death. For comparison, Figure 1(a) is in color and Figure 1(b) in black and white.

The lines on a contour map connect adjacent points on a surface that are of equal height; these lines are sometimes called level lines or isograms. In Figure 1, one of the level lines represents a probability of death of about 3.85%: the line starts in 1886 at age 64 and ends in 1986 at age 70, indicating that 70-year-old Italian men in the 1980s faced the same chance of mortality as 64-year-olds faced a century earlier.

All demographic data pertain to discrete intervals of age and time. Demographic rates and probabilities typically pertain to squares, rectangles or trapezoids on the age-time plane. The LEXISMAP computer program plots such data to represent the underlying nature of the data: the mortality surface is tiled with small discrete areas. An alternative strategy is to assure that the value for each discrete area equals the value at the point in the "center" of the area. Then, a smooth surface could be estimated by interpolation, and sinuous contour lines could be drawn. This approach was adopted in our earlier LEXIS software; similar contour-map algorithms are used in several other software packages. We now prefer the discrete-area strategy because it reveals the underlying nature of the demographic data being mapped.

The major features of the evolution of Italian male mortality are apparent on the map. The devastation of World War I and the Spanish influenza epidemic appears as a

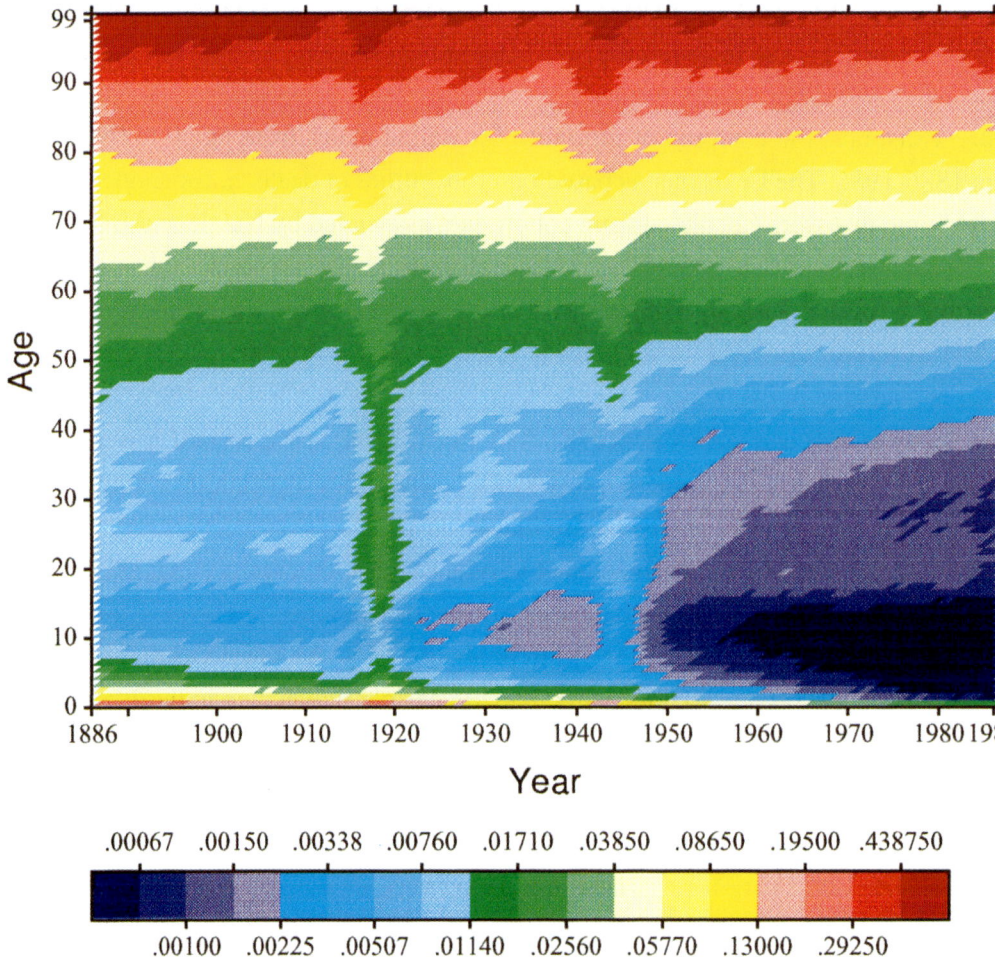

**Figure 1(a).** Probabilities of death for Italian males (in color), with contours from 0.00067 to 0.43875 at multiples of 1.5, and from age 0 to 99 and year 1886 to 1986.

sharp ridge of high mortality that interrupts the map around 1918. A lower ridge shows the effects of World War II. The general pattern over time is one of progress against mortality, rapid at younger ages and slower at advanced ages. The general pattern over age is equally clear: high mortality in infancy and again among the elderly. The intriguing diagonal patterns suggest possible cohort effects, most notably during the 1920s and 1930s among the cohorts born around 1900: males in these cohorts, who were in their late teens and early 20s during World War I, may have been particularly debilitated by the war and its aftermath. Also notable are the various islands and peninsulas of high mortality that run across the map between ages 20 and 25: as discussed by Caselli et al. (1985a,b), these reflect various disruptive socioeconomic and political events in Italian history as well as the tendency for younger men to engage in reckless behavior.

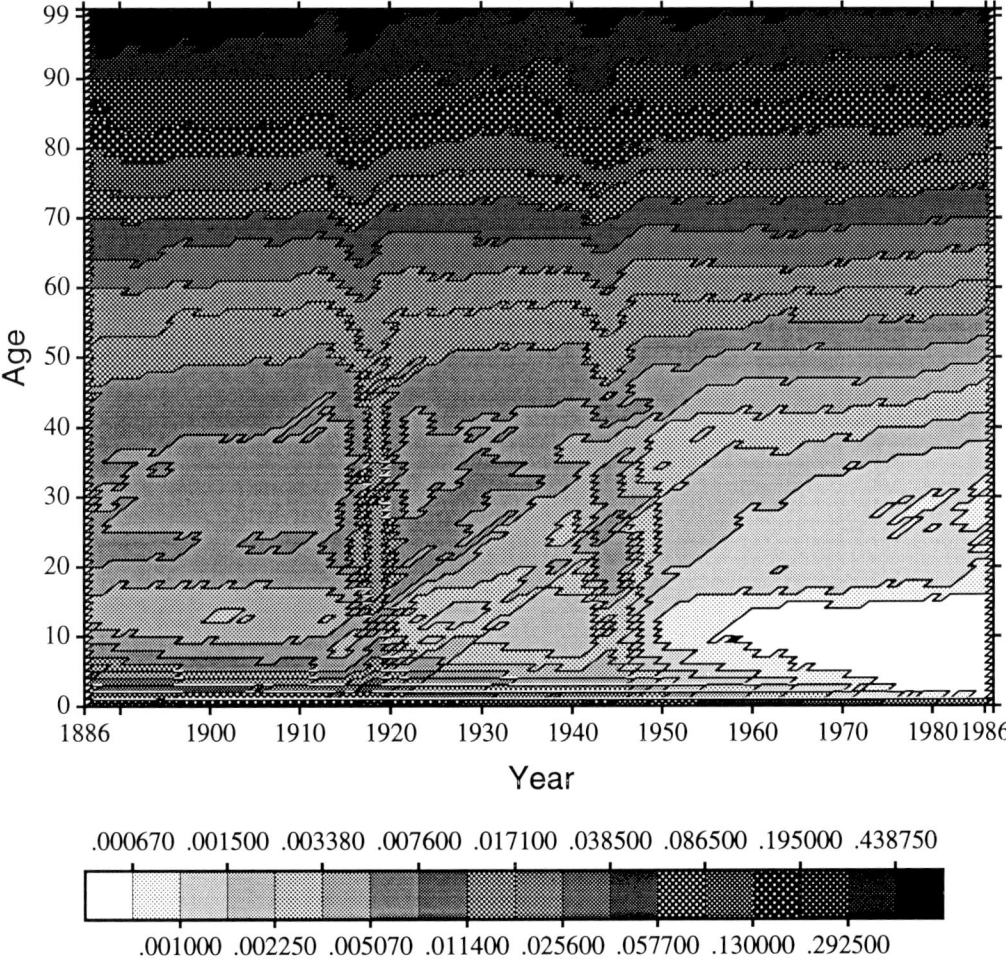

**Figure 1(b).** Probabilities of death for Italian males (in black and white), with contour lines from 0.00067 to 0.43875 at multiples of 1.5, and from age 0 to 99 and year 1886 to 1986.

# 3. Levels, shades, and grids

An important consideration when designing a contour map is how many different levels to use. The LEXISMAP computer program that we employed to draw the maps allows, among other possibilities, lines to be drawn at 17 levels, separating the surface into 18 tiers. Use of fewer lines sacrifices detail, whereas use of more lines tends to make the map less intelligible: 17 levels is a reasonable compromise, although the use of 10 or 20 levels might be considered. Delaporte (1941) draws lines at 19, 20, or 21 levels on his various maps of European mortality; many of the figures in this monograph use fewer than 17 levels. Figure 1(c) presents the contours of Italian male mortality using 10 levels rather than the 17 levels used in Figure 1(b).

Which specific elevations the contour lines should connect is a second important design decision. On mortality surfaces, where probabilities might approach a minimum of the order of magnitude of 0.0001 and a maximum of 1, use of equally spaced lines-say at 0.01, 0.02, and so on up to 0.15-results in a map where the contours are clumped together at the youngest and oldest ages, with a largely empty expanse in-between. Figure 1(d) illustrates this for Italian male mortality. The map is far more informative when the lines are spread out at constant multiples-e.g., each line representing a level 50% higher than the previous line, as in Figure 1(b). Alternatively, a convenient scale can be used: Delaporte places his lines at levels of mortality of 1, 2, 3, ..., 9, 10, 12, 15, 20, 30, 50, 100, 150, 200, 250, 300, 350, and 400 per thousand, and in several figures in this monograph, including Figures 5 and 17, contour lines are selectively placed at convenient levels.

Shifting the location of contour lines can make a difference in the appearance of a Lexis map, especially in the details. The map in Figure 1(e) provides an example. Compare, for instance, the region from 1920 to 1930 from age 20 to 30 on Figure 1(b) and (e).

Demographers often work with transformations, such as the log or logit, so it might seem reasonable to transform the surface $q(x,y)$ into the surface of, say, $\log q(x,y)$ and then to draw level lines at equal intervals on the transformed surface. If the transformation is monotonic, like the log or logit transformation, an identical contour map can be drawn by spacing the level lines at appropriately unequal intervals on the original surface. In the case of logarithms, the level lines should be multiples of each other rather than being equally spaced. Thus, the map in, say, Figure 1(a) can also be interpreted as depicting log probabilities of death.

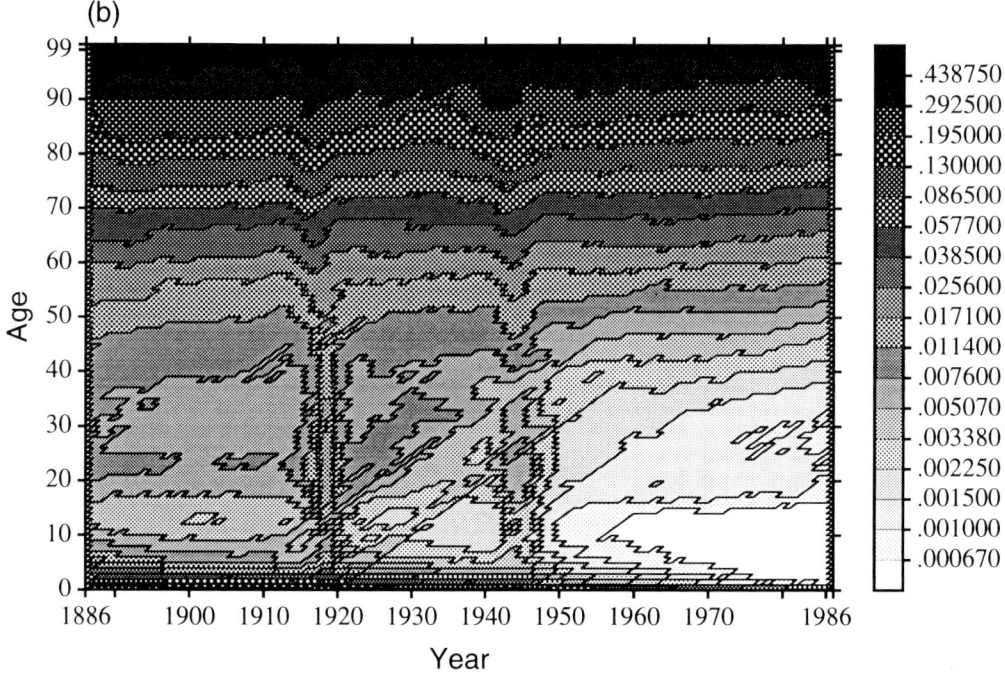

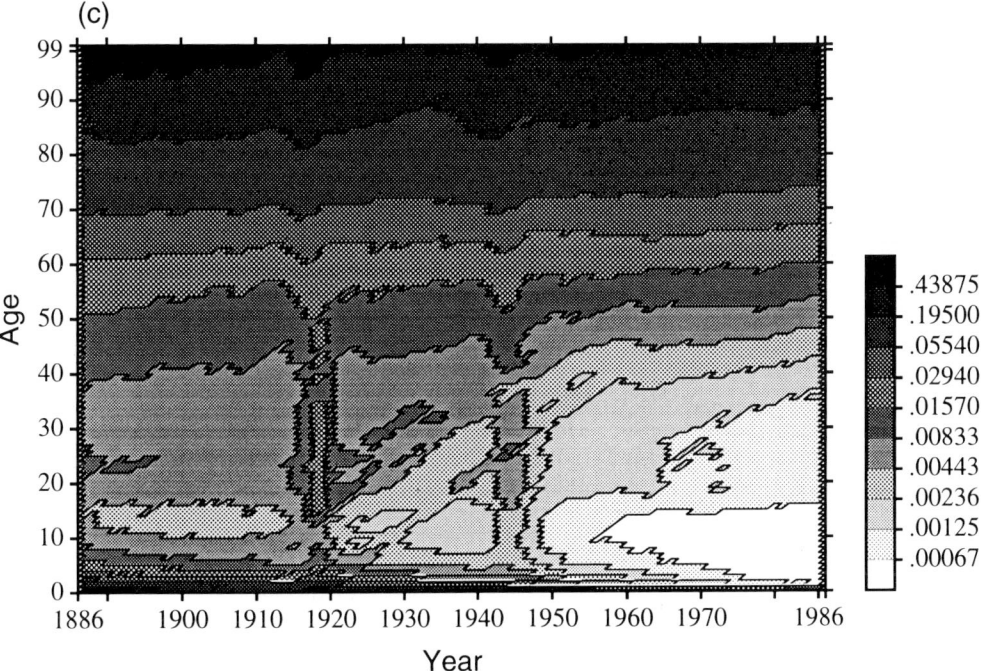

**Figure 1(c).** Probabilities of death for Italian males: (b) (repeated) with contour lines from 0.00067 to 0.43875 at multiples of 1.5, and from age 0 to 99 and year 1886 to 1986; (c) as Figure 1(b), but with 10 contour lines from 0.00067 to 0.43875.

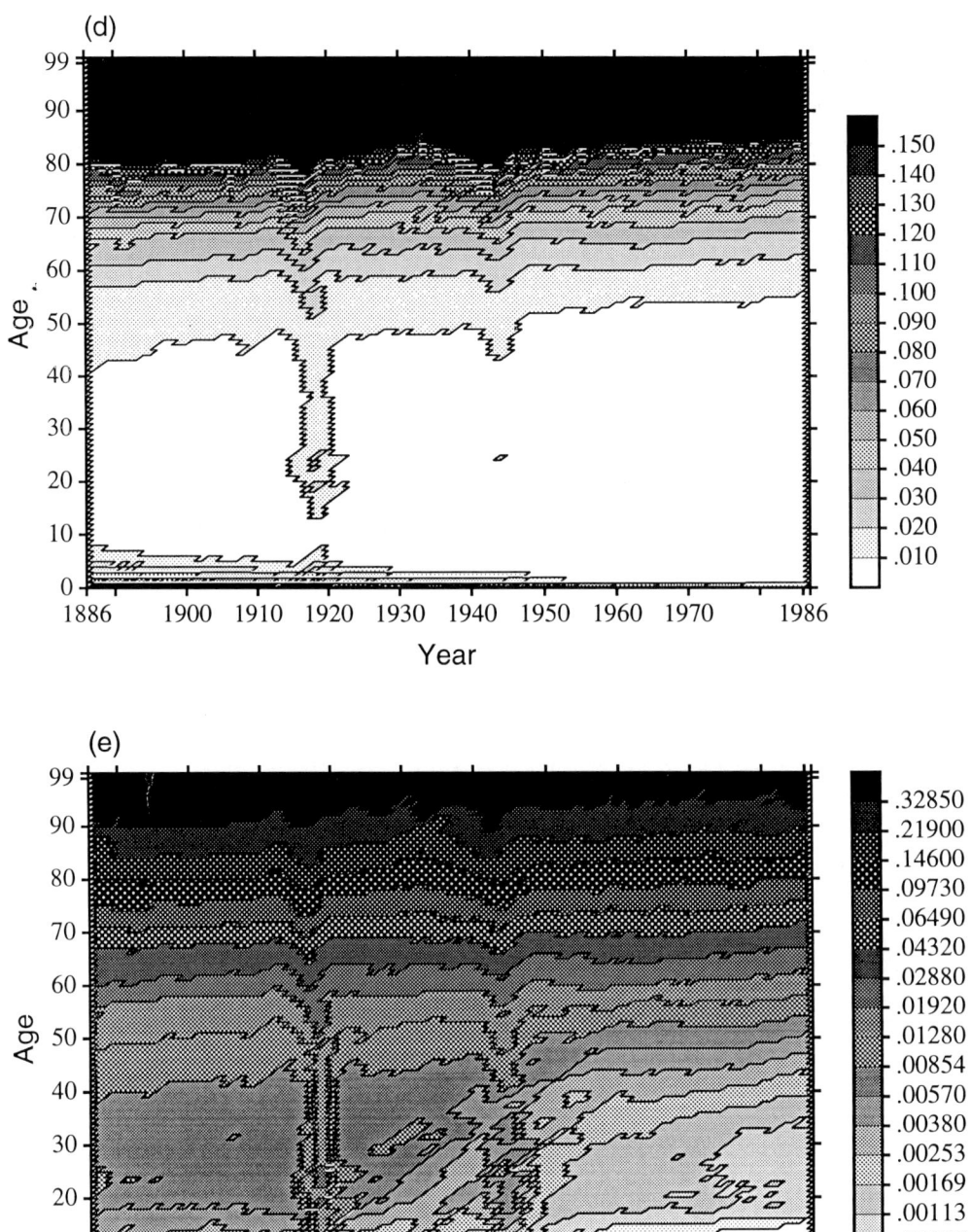

**Figure 1(d,e).** Probabilities of death for Italian males: (d) as Figure 1(b), but with evenly spaced contour lines from 0.01 to 0.15; (e) as Figure 1(b), but with 17 contour lines starting at 0.0005.

A key feature of the LEXISMAP computer program we developed is the shading of regions according to the height of the surface. The shading varies from light to dark or from deep purple to deep red as the surfaces rise from low to high levels of mortality. Such shading, which is time-consuming to do by hand but easy with the help of a computer, makes the overall pattern of a mortality surface more immediately comprehensible, especially if the map is viewed at a distance. At the same time, the details of small peaks and pits and of the twists and turns of the contour lines are still there to be scrutinized at close range. Literature, critics note, can be profitably read at different levels of understanding; we suggest that the reader try viewing Figure 1(a) and perhaps some of the other figures in this monograph at levels of 25 cm and 5 m.

Sometimes it is useful to draw a grid on a contour map so that the coordinates of various points can be conveniently located. In Figure 1(f) the map in Figure 1(b) is redrawn with a superimposed grid every 20 years of time and age. The grid detracts a bit from the underlying pattern-that is the price of adding additional information. Grids are also included in Figures 2(a), 2(b), and 28.

To see general trends it may be helpful to suppress the contour lines in a map of a population surface. In Figure 1(g) the map in Figure 1(b) is redrawn with shading but without lines. Alternatively, one could draw a conditional contour map with lines but without shading. Figure 1(h) displays such a map for Italian male mortality. The lines in this figure are not labelled, but they could be.

# 4. Smoothed maps

It is useful to take a close look at the small blemishes isolated from contour lines on a Lexis map, because these spots indicate outliers-very localized peaks or pits-that might be due to erroneous data values. Consider, for instance, the black rhombus in the first graph of Figure 1(b) at age 9 and year 1957: it turns out that this blemish was, indeed, produced by an error made in transcribing the Italian mortality data to a computer tape. (The error was corrected, but we have left the spot as an illustration). On the other hand, the mark at age 19 in 1962 represents a point where the mortality surface barely crosses a contour level, like the top of a sea mount that appears as a small island just rising above the level of the surrounding ocean.

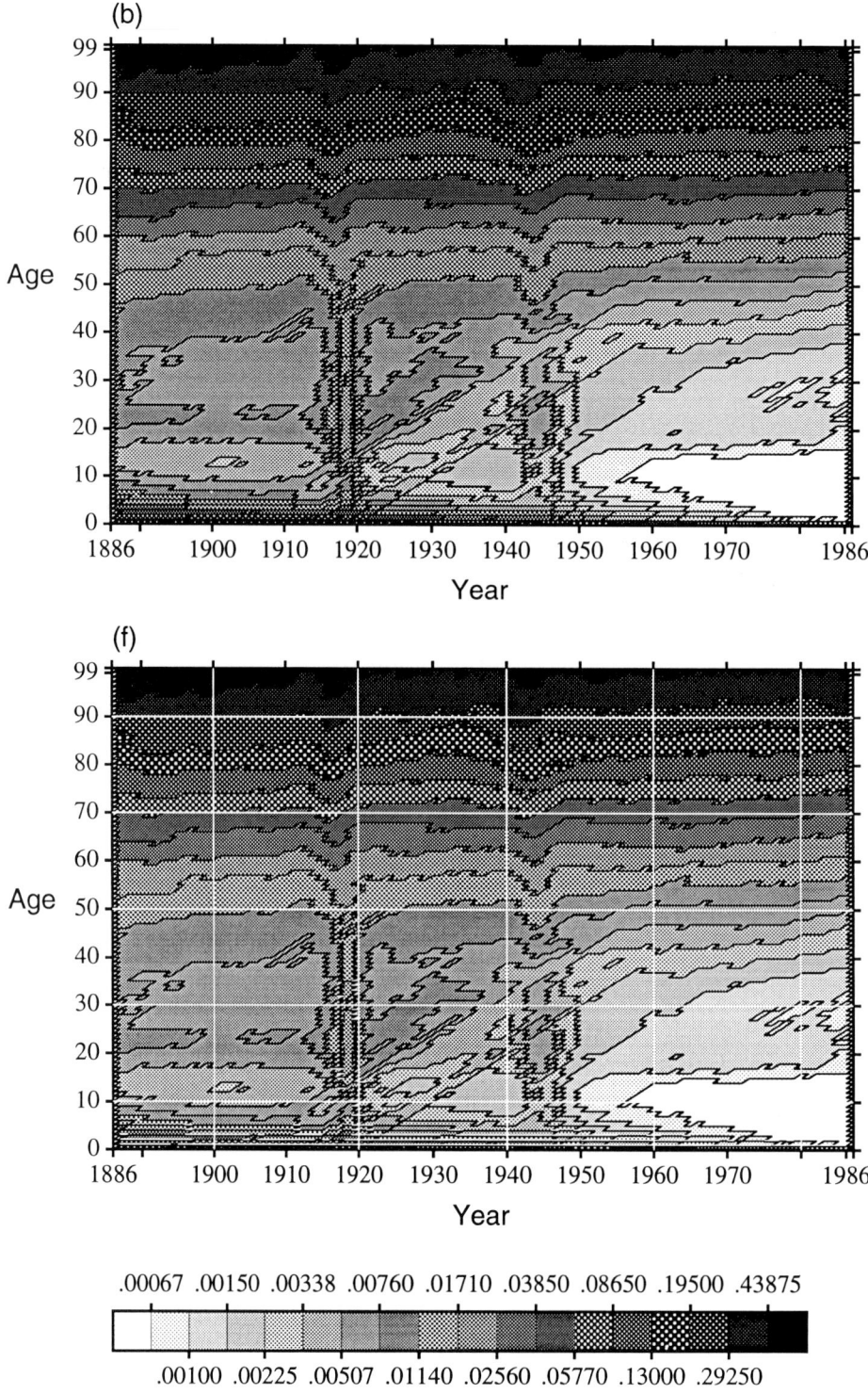

**Figure 1(f).** Probabilities of death for Italian males: (b) (repeated) with contour lines from 0.00067 to 0.43875 at multiples of 1.5, and from age 0 to 99 and year 1886 to 1986; (f) as Figure 1(b), but with grid.

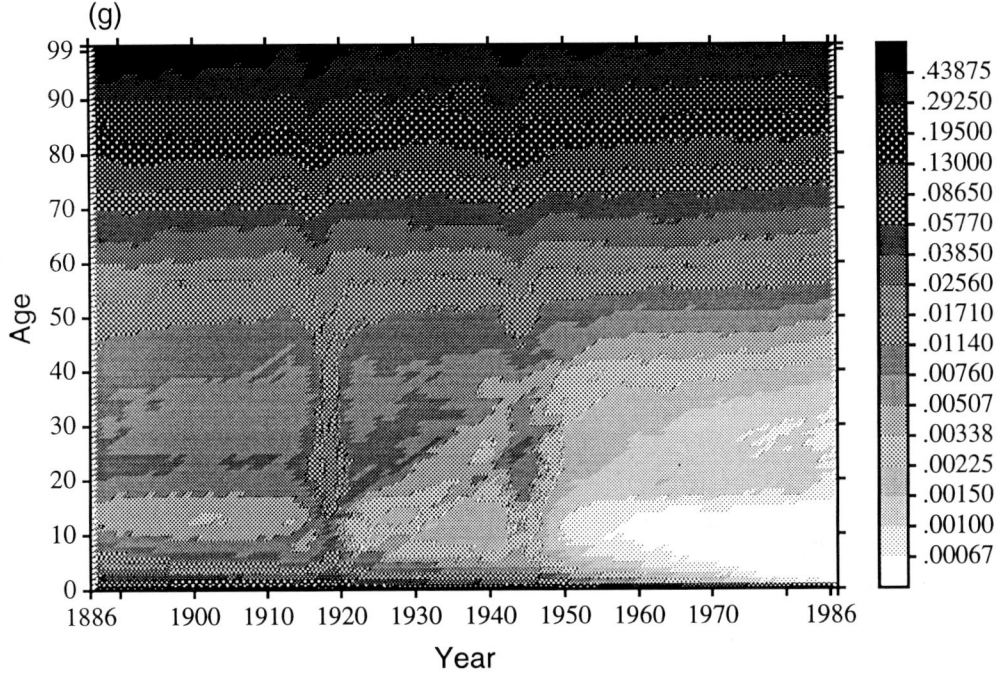

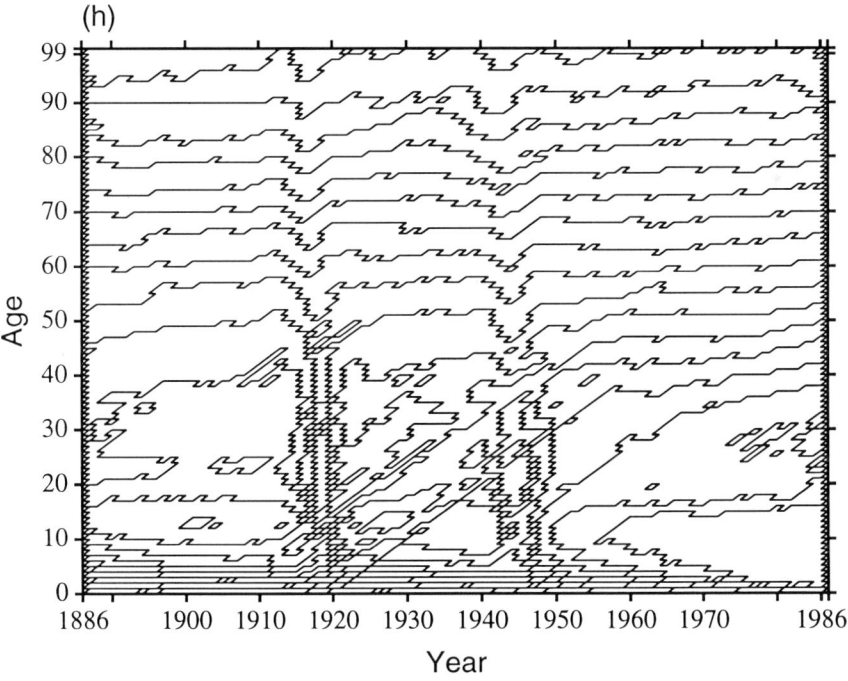

**Figure 1(g,h).** Probabilities of death for Italian males: (g) as Figure 1(b), but without contour lines; (h) as Figure 1(b), but without shading.

In addition to these blemishes, some cluttered areas appear in Figure 1(b). These represent virtual plateaus where the mortality surface is repeatedly crossing and recrossing a level line, or cliffs where mortality rates are rising or falling rapidly. To reduce this kind of noise and to suppress the details of local fluctuations so that the global patterns can be more clearly perceived, it may be useful to smooth a surface. Delaporte (1941) presented both raw and smoothed contour maps of mortality in various European countries: on his "adjusted" maps, he drew smooth contour lines based on his feeling for the data. We used a mechanistic, computer algorithm to produce the smoothed map shown in Figure 1(i). In the smoothed map the height of the surface at age $x$ in year $y$ was replaced by the average of the 25 heights in the 5 x 5 square of points from $(x - 2)$ to $(x + 2)$ and from $(y - 2)$ to $(y + 2)$. On the edges of the map, where a full 5 x 5 array of data points is not available, the smoothing procedure averages the available data.

Instead of smoothing by averaging over a 5 x 5 square, a larger (or smaller) square might be used. In Figure 1(j) Italian male mortality is smoothed on an 11 x 11 square. Global patterns in this map are somewhat clearer than in Figure 1(i), but some interesting local detail is lost and effects that are concentrated in time or age, such as infant mortality and mortality during the 1918 Spanish influenza epidemic, are smeared out.

A variety of alternative smoothing procedures might be used, including procedures that replace points by a weighted average of adjacent points, the weights diminishing with distance. Figure 1(k) presents a map of Italian male mortality smoothed by an algorithm in which the weights given to the points in a 5 x 5 square were proportional to the matrix:

$$\begin{matrix} 1 & 4 & 6 & 4 & 1 \\ 4 & 16 & 24 & 16 & 4 \\ 6 & 24 & 36 & 24 & 6 \\ 4 & 16 & 24 & 16 & 4 \\ 1 & 4 & 6 & 4 & 1 \end{matrix}$$

Thus, the points in the corners of the square were given weights of 1/256, whereas the point in the center received a weight of 36/256. The theoretical advantages of such weighted smoothing algorithms (see Tukey (1977) for an introductory discussion) have to be balanced against the conceptual simplicity and computational convenience of the kind of straightforward averaging illustrated in Figures 1(j) and 1(k).

By using fewer contour lines, a less busy and hence smoother-looking Lexis map can usually be produced. Figure 1(l) illustrates of an extreme example of this approach: Italian male mortality is represented on a Lexis map on which all but three of the contours (and four of the levels) have been suppressed. The map, in its simplicity, strikingly highlights the rapid progress against mortality at younger ages, especially after World War II, in contrast with the slower progress at older ages.

# 5. Close-ups

As mentioned above and as discussed by Caselli et al. (1985a), the patterns of male mortality in Italy from ages 10 to 49 for years 1910 to 1969 reveal some interesting cohort effects. Figures 2(a) and 2(b) present Lexis maps of this restricted age and time area: the maps can be considered as enlargements or close-ups of a section of the map in Figure 1(b). Thus, contour maps can be used both to display a large data array and also to focus on selected portions of the array. Note that because in Figure 2(a) the contours are drawn at the same levels as in the original Figure 1(b), only half of the possible levels are utilized. In Figure 2(b), twice as many contours are drawn as in Figure 2(a), every other contour in the second figure being at the same level as a contour in the first figure. Part of the advantage of a close-up is that if the height of the surface varies less in the restricted region being scrutinized, then the level lines can be located at closer intervals to reveal more local detail.

Figures 2(a) and 2(b) make the diagonal patterns on Figure 1(b) more apparent; the added grid makes it clear that the patterns do, indeed, run along cohort lines. Consider one of the most striking differences on the map, the difference between the mortality rates suffered by the cohort born in 1903 and the cohort born in 1908. These two cohort diagonals are separated at most ages between 10 and 30 by two contour levels, indicating a rough mortality differential of about 50%; after age 30 the discrepancy appears to sharply diminish and then disappear.

To explore this intriguing differential and similar differentials among nearby cohorts, we produced Figure 2(c), which plots contour lines of mortality for the cohorts born between 1894 and 1924; these cohorts are followed from age 0 to 54. Note that in Figure 2(c), year of birth runs along the horizontal axis, not current year. The figure reveals some strong cohort differences, especially among cohorts born between 1903 and

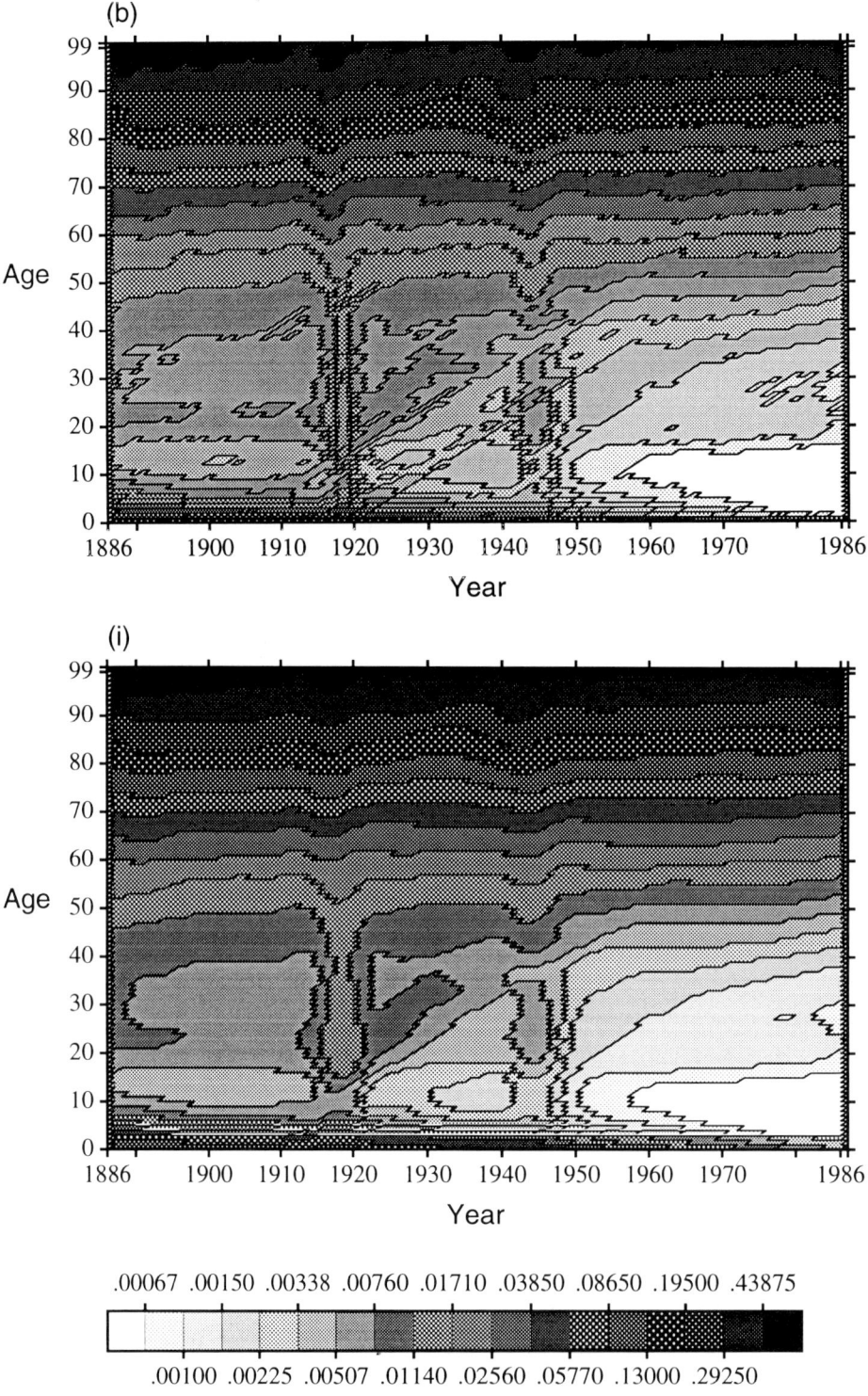

**Figure 1(i).** Probabilities of death for Italian males: (b) (repeated) with contour lines from 0.00067 to 0.43875 at multiples of 1.5, and from age 0 to 99 and year 1886 to 1986; (i) as Figure 1(b), but smoothed on a 5 x 5 square.

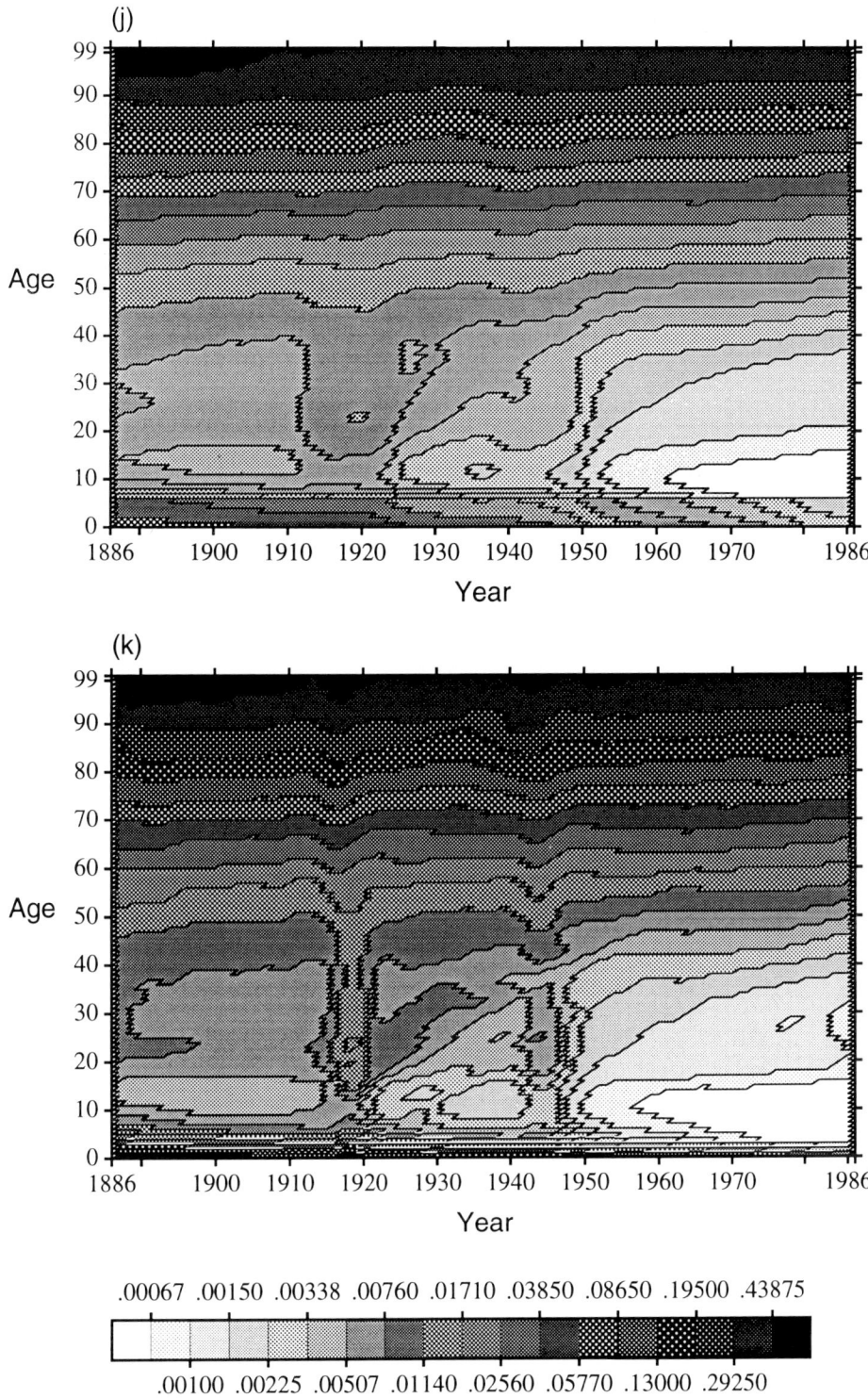

**Figure 1(j,k).** Probabilities of death for Italian males: (j) as Figure 1(b), but smoothed on a 11 x 11 square; (k) as Figure 1(b), but smoothed on a weighted 5 x 5 square.

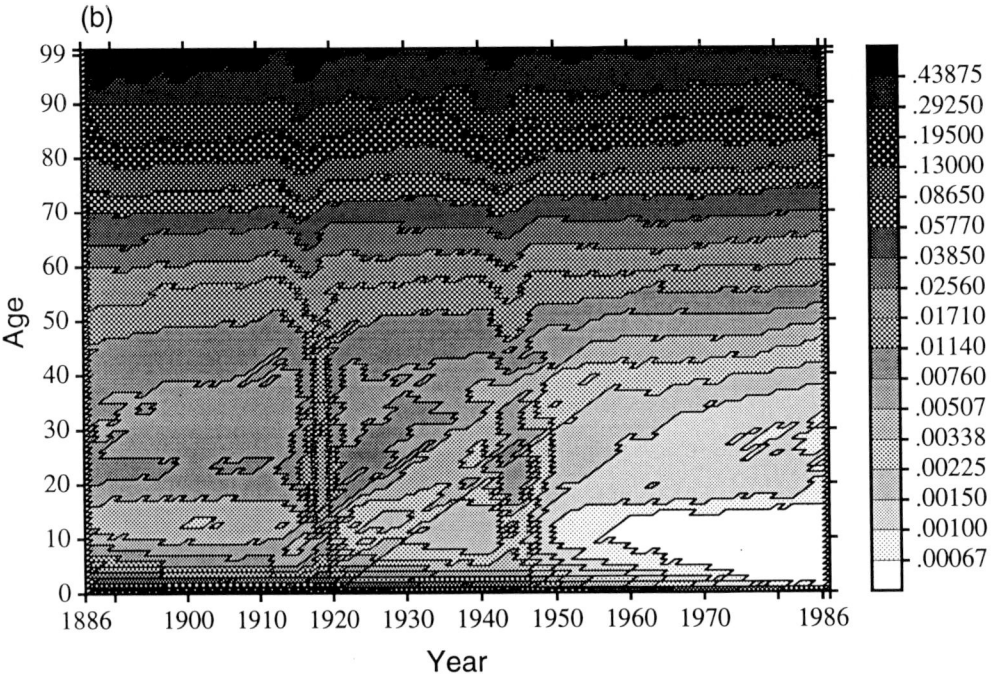

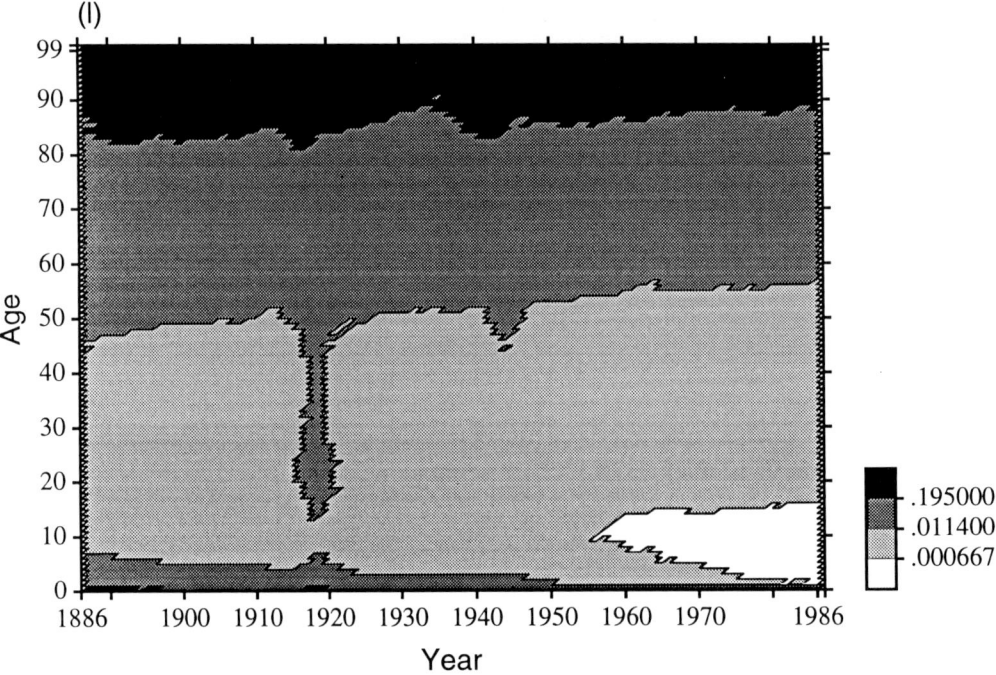

**Figure 1(l).** Probabilities of death for Italian males: (b)(repeated) with contour lines from 0.00067 to 0.43875 at multiples of 1.5, and from age 0 to 99 and year 1886 to 1986; (l) as Figure 1(b), but with only three contour lines.

1909 and among cohorts born between 1917 and 1920. It is interesting to see how the period effects of World Wars I and II appear on this figure, as backward diagonals.

To more closely scrutinize the differences among the cohorts born between 1903 and 1909, we produced Figure 2(d), which plots the contours of the mortality rates experienced by the 1904 to 1909 cohorts, from age 0 to age 54, relative to the mortality rates experienced by the 1903 cohort. Thus, Figure 2(d) facilitates comparisons of the cohorts, with the 1903 cohort serving as the standard for comparison. In the case of the 1908 cohort, for instance, the map reveals that the 1903 cohort suffered substantially higher mortality at all ages except ages 8, 9, and 10. The 1903 cohort experienced these ages just prior to the First World War, whereas the 1908 cohort passed through these ages during the final years of the war and the Spanish Influenza epidemic. At ages 14 and 15, which the 1903 cohort lived through from 1917 to 1919, the 1903 cohort experienced more than five times the mortality experienced at these same ages by the 1908 cohort. Rough calculations indicate that between ages 16 and 34, mortality rates for the 1908 cohort averaged about 50% of those for the 1903 cohort, and between ages 35 and 54 mortality rates were about 30% lower on average.

Thus, the general tendency was for the risk differential to diminish, but local fluctuations complicate the pattern. Careful scrutiny of the details of the pattern of mortality differential between the 1903 and 1908 cohorts, and of similar differentials between other cohorts, might lead to better understanding of the interaction of age, period and cohort effects. More generally, our use of Figures 1(b) and 2(a)-2(d) provides a suggestive illustration of the value of contour maps in exploratory analyses of population surfaces.

# 6. Maps from interpolated data

The mortality statistics for Italian males used in Figures 1 and 2 are available by single year of age and single year of time, i.e. year of birth. Frequently, demographers have to work with less finely-spaced data; death rates, for instance, may be available every decade or so, by five-year age classes. Figure 3(a) displays the evolution of Italian male mortality based on data published in Preston et al. (1972). Data sets from this source were available for 1881, 1891, 1901, 1910, 1921, 1931, 1960, and 1964. Probabilities of death were given for five-year age categories from age 5 up to age 80, as well as for ages 0 and

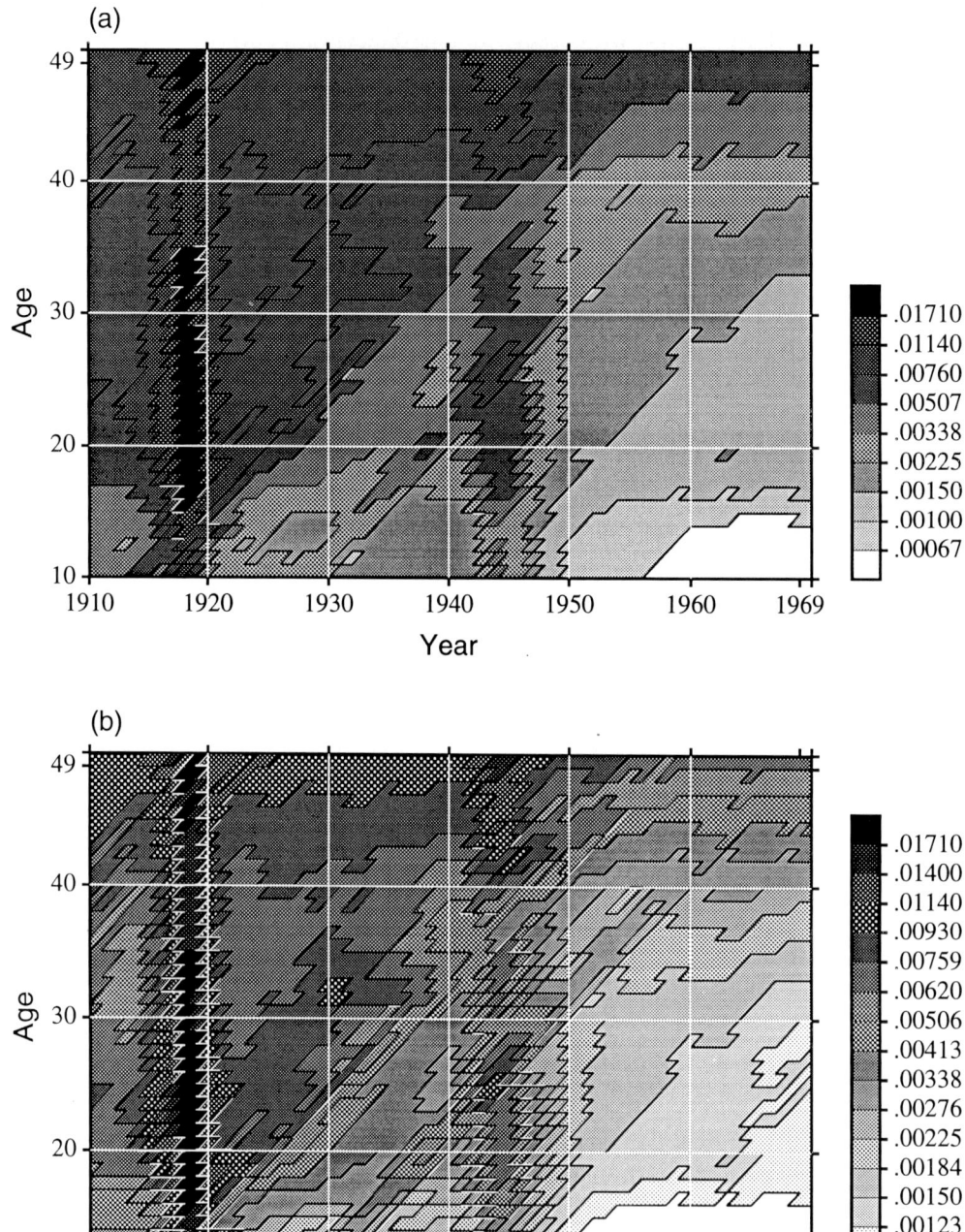

**Figure 2(a,b).** Probabilities of death for Italian males: (a) with a grid, contour lines from 0.00067 to 0.0171 at multiples of 1.5, and from age 10 to 49 and year 1910 to 1969; (b) with a grid, contour lines from 0.00100 to 0.0171 at multiples of square root of 1.5, and from age 10 to 49 and year 1910 to 1969.

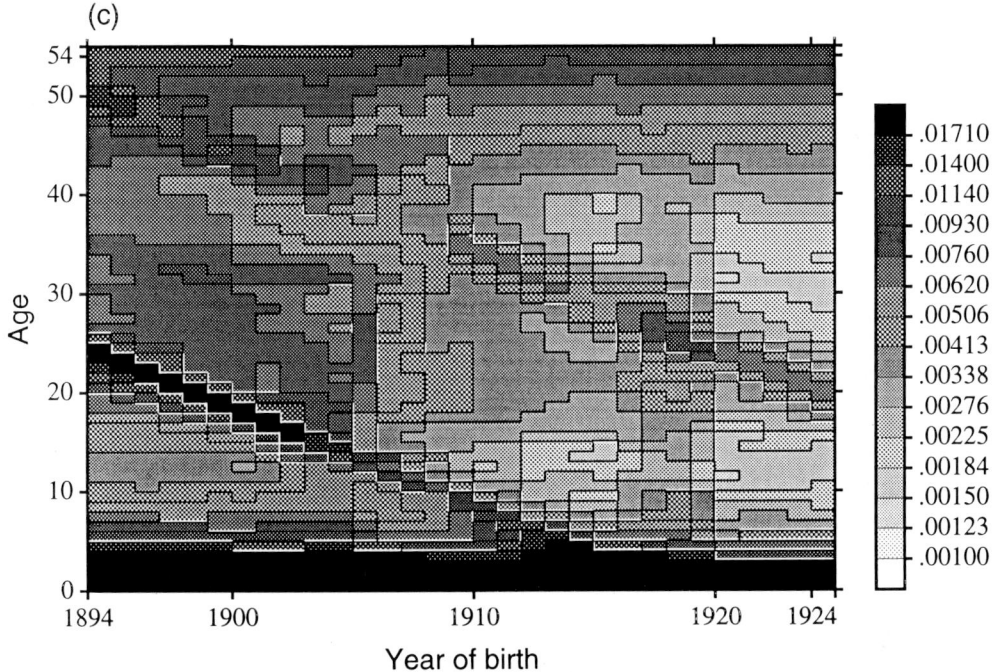

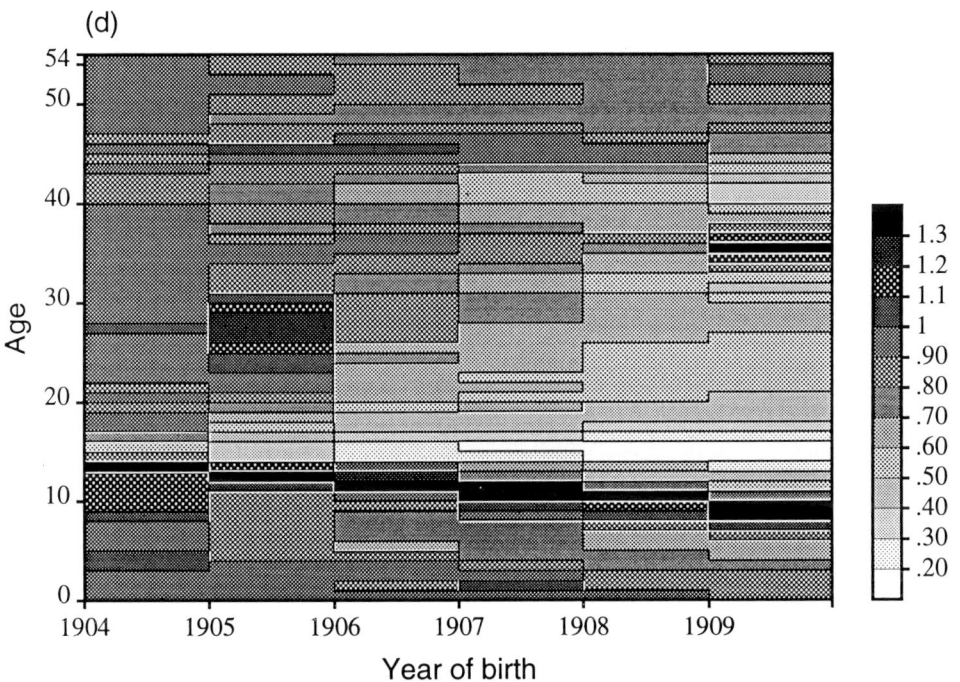

**Figure 2(c,d).** (c) Probabilities of death for cohorts of Italian males, with a grid, contour lines from 0.00100 to 0.0171 at multiples of square root of 1.5, and from age 0 to 54 and year of birth 1894 to 1924. (d) Probabilities of death for Italian males relative to 1903 cohort age-specific levels, with contour lines from 0.2 to 1.3 at intervals of 0.1, and from age 0 to 54 and year of birth 1904 to 1909.

38

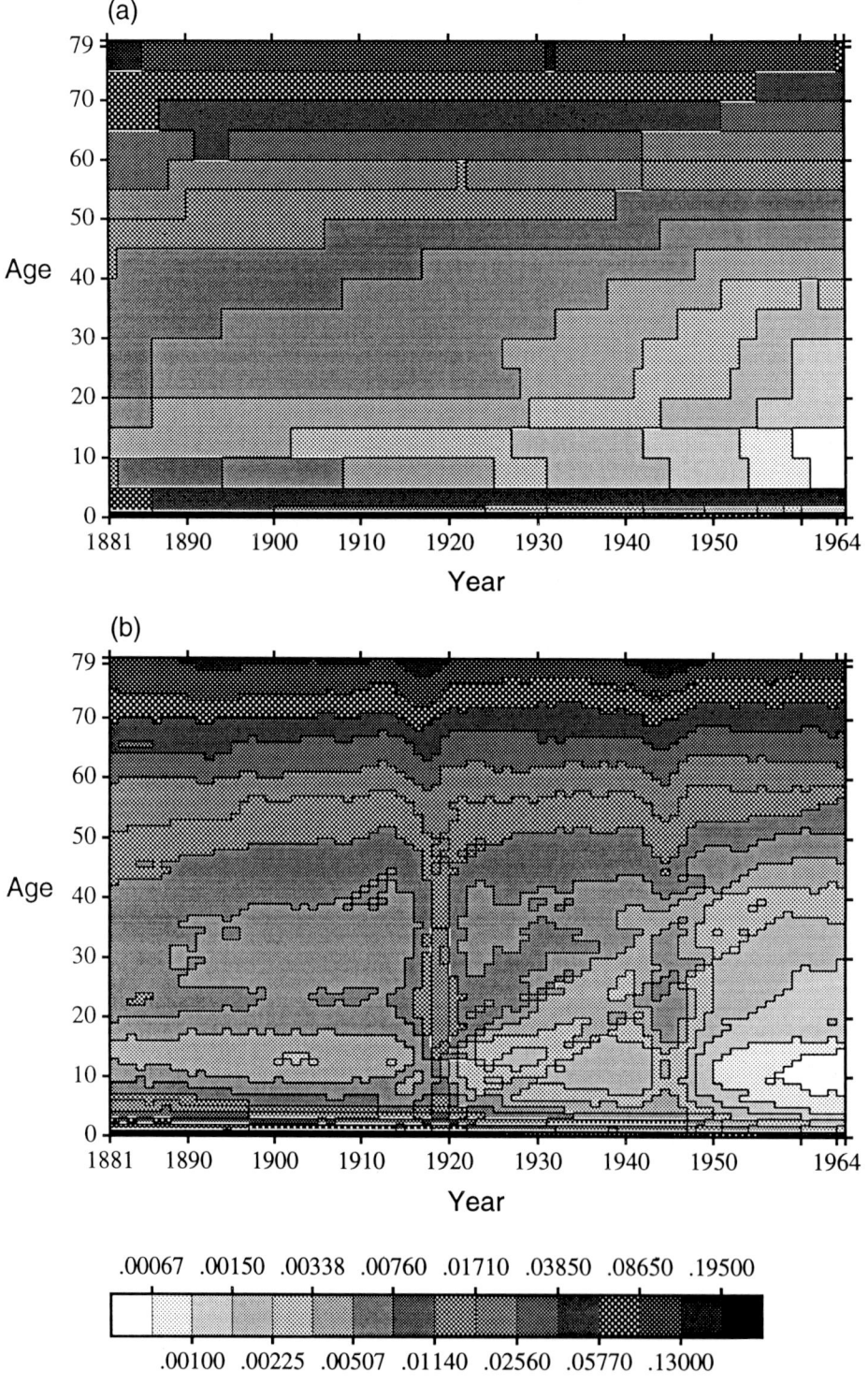

**Figure 3.** Probabilities of death for Italian males, with contour lines from 0.00067 to 0.195 at multiples of 1.5, and from age 0 to 79 and year 1881 to 1964.
(a) interpolated data; (b) single-year-of-time-and-age data.

1 and the three-year category from age 2 to 5. We converted the n-year statistics into single-year statistics such that the resulting mortality curve followed a piece-wise linear trajectory; we then used simple linear interpolation between the available data points over time to estimate the height of the mortality surface at intermediate points in time. Comparison of Figures 3(a) and 3(b), which presents single-year of age and time data at the same scale, reveals the difference between working with detailed data and interpolated data. The global patterns of mortality over age and time are apparent in Figure 3(a), but all the interesting local features, including the effects of World Wars I and II, are lost.

The longest time series of mortality statistics are available for Sweden. We used probabilities of death based on interpolations made by Vaupel et al. (1979) and, for recent years, by ourselves, of data from Keyfitz and Flieger (1968) for 1778 to 1882 and from

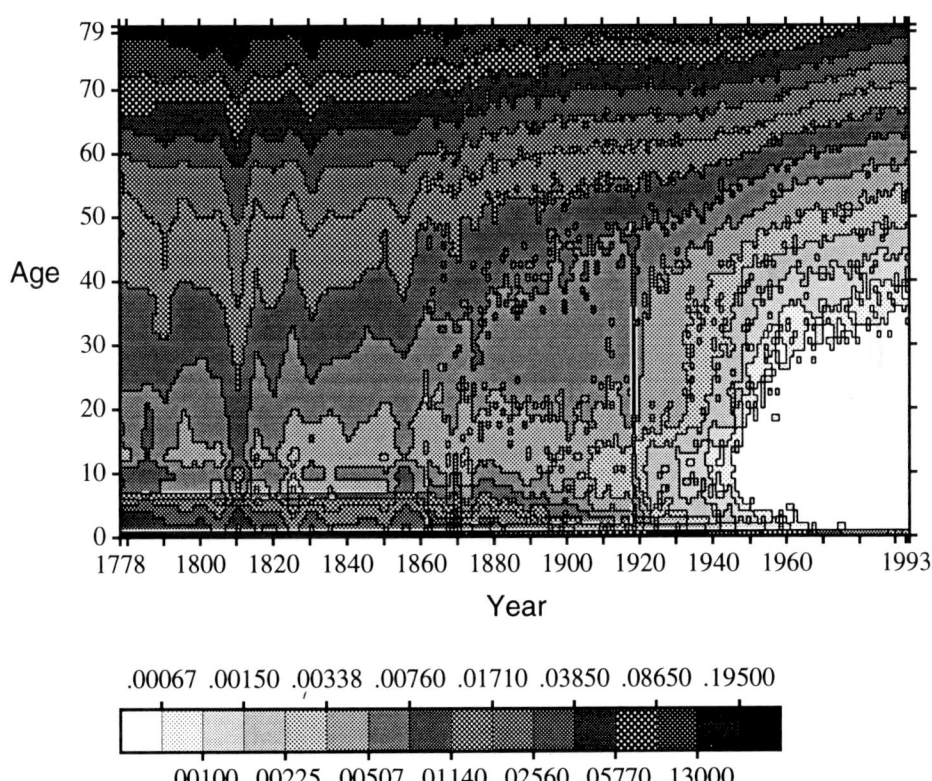

**Figure 4.** Probabilities of death for Swedish females, with contour lines from 0.00067 to 0.195 at multiples of 1.5, and from age 0 to 79 and year 1778 to 1993.

various editions of the Swedish Statistical Yearbook from 1881 on. These data were available for the most part for five year periods; before 1880 the data were given for five year age categories but thereafter data by single year of age were available. It is apparent from Figure 4 which shows the evolution of Swedish female mortality from 1779 to 1993 that systematic progress against mortality at all ages began in Sweden around 1830. A remarkable acceleration of progress, especially at younger ages, starts after 1920. In early years, strong fluctuations are evident, especially the destructive effects of the Swedish war with Russia in 1808-1809.

# 7. Maps of female fertility

Figure 5 displays the contours of US birth rates from 1917 to 1990 for women from age 14 to 49; the figure is based on data compiled by Heuser (1976, 1984). In the center of the baby boom, for women around age 23 around 1960, fully a quarter of women gave birth each year. The concentration of high birth rates among women in their early- and mid-20s and the cycles of high and low birth rates that characterize baby booms and busts are strikingly revealed on the map. The color scale in Figure 5 was chosen to allow comparison with Chinese and Finnish birth rates in Figures 8 and 9.

Figure 5 is a standard map in which current year runs along the horizontal axis and age runs up the vertical axis. Other coordinates help reveal cohort effects. In particular, because the eye can follow vertical and horizontal lines more easily than diagonals, it may be useful to twist a contour map so that year of birth, rather than current year, runs along the horizontal axis, as in Figures 6 and 7. Fewer contour lines are plotted in Figure 7 because the lines were otherwise too closely spaced to be intelligible.

Taken together, Figures 5, 6, and 7 indicate that the age effect in fertility is very strong, that period fluctuations are also strong, but that cohort effects appear to be much less prominent. Perhaps more refined methods of presentation will reveal persistent cohort patterns; some relevant analysis is presented later in this monograph in conjunction with Figures 10, 11, 15, 18 through 20, 27, and 40. Note that the period effects shown in Figures 5, 6, and 7 can be separated into three parts. Before age 18, birth rates have remained low, and after age 35 or so, there is a general pattern of declining

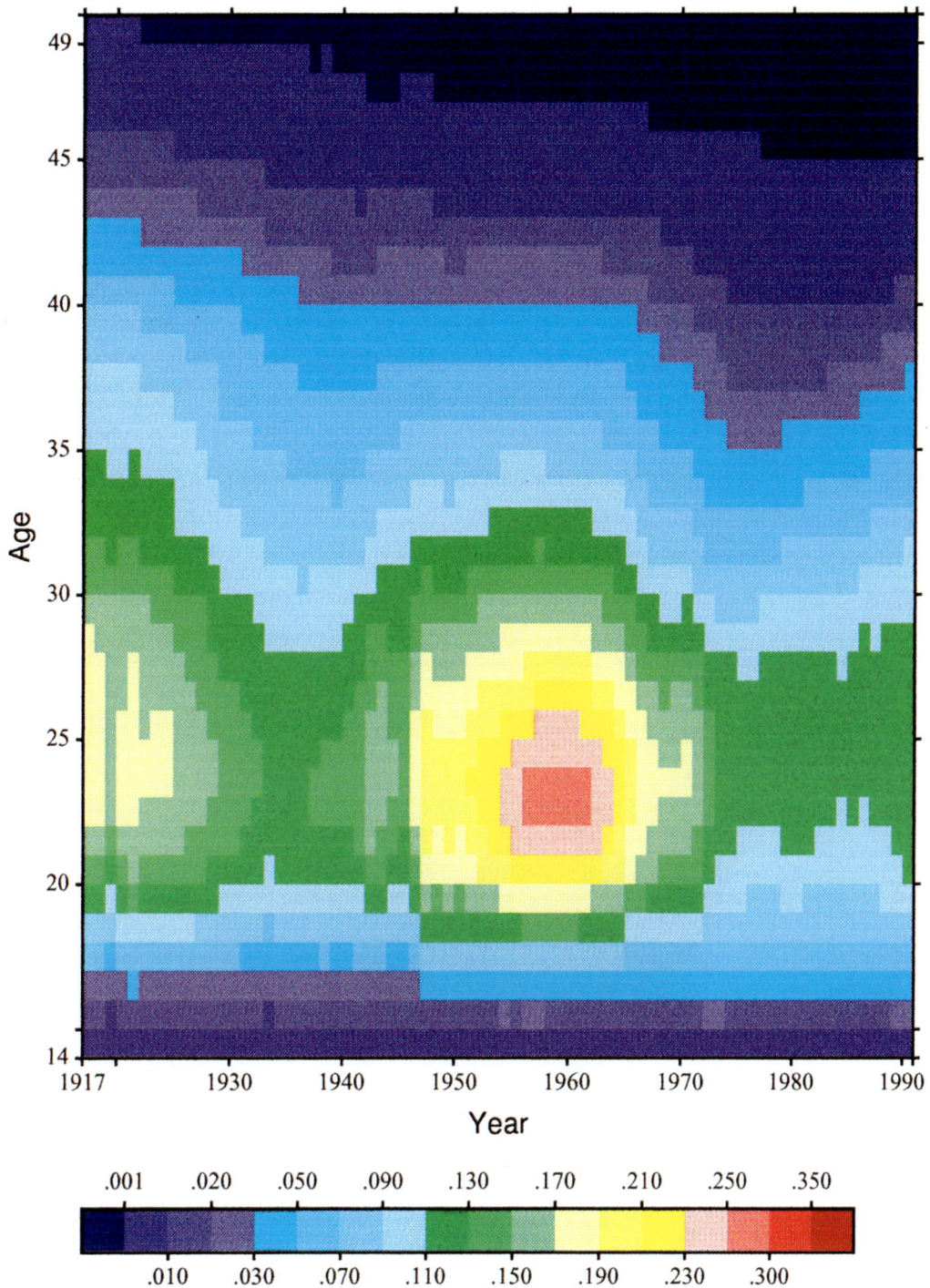

**Figure 5.** US birth rates, with contours selectively placed from 0.001 to 0.35, and from age 14 to 49 and year 1917 to 1990.

fertility up until the late 1970s. It is between ages 18 and 35, and especially around age 23, where the most dramatic absolute swings in fertility have occurred. In conjunction with Figure 15, we will consider relative fluctuations in birth rates, in contrast with absolute fluctuations shown in Figures 5, 6, and 7.

Figure 8 displays a Lexis map of Chinese birth rates by single year of age from 15 to 49 and single year of time from 1940 to 1989; the map is presented and discussed in Zeng et al. (1985, 1994). As discussed in those articles, the most striking feature of the map is the rapid decline in fertility during the 1970s. This decline is well known and often summarized by the dramatic drop in the total fertility rate: in 1970 the total fertility rate was 5.8; by 1981 it had fallen 55% to 2.6. What the map graphically reveals is the age pattern of decline. Consider the ages where the birth rate exceeds 20%: in 1968, this period of high fertility stretched from age 20 through 37. By 1981, in contrast, the period of high fertility was concentrated from age 23 to 27. In 1968, more than 20% of 20-year-olds and more than 10% of 40-year-olds gave birth. By 1981, the birth rate of 20-year-olds had fallen under 10% and the birth rate of 40-year-olds had fallen under 2%. The precipitous decline in the fertility contours at older ages and the marked increase in the

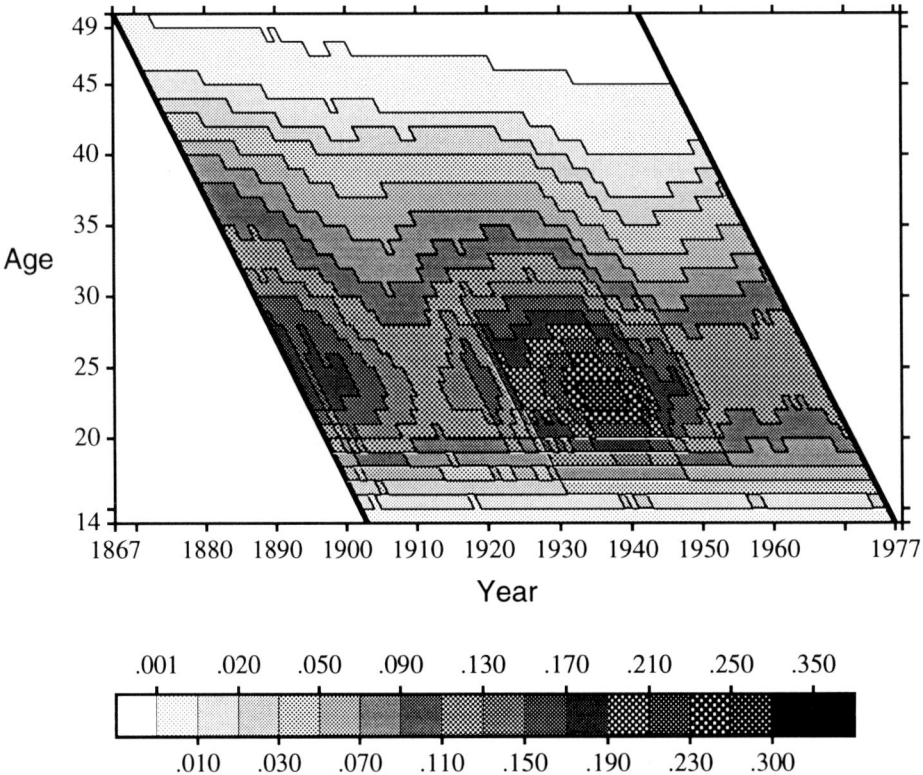

**Figure 6.** US cohort birth rates, with contour lines selectively placed from 0.001 to 0.35, and from age 14 to 49 and year of birth 1867 to 1977.

contours at younger ages reflect the success of Chinese birth control policy, including the increase in age of first marriage (cf. Figure 29) and, even more importantly, the widespread use of contraception.

The radical narrowing of the period of high fertility was slightly reversed in 1981. Since then, birth rates have remained roughly the same, albeit with some shift to greater fertility at ages 20 - 24. This is partially a result of the New Marriage Law, announced in 1980, and the concomitant boom in marriages, especially among women in their mid-20s.

The most conspicuous period disruption on the map is the trough in fertility in 1959-1961. This coincides with the Great Leap Forward and corresponds to a similar trough in marriage rates, except that marriage rates tended to be lowest in 1959 whereas fertility rates reached their low point in 1961. The recovery of birth rates from their depressed level in 1961 was dramatic: during the prolific ages between 23 and 29, birth rates rose from about 20% per year in 1961 to over 30% per year in 1962 and over 35% per year in 1963.

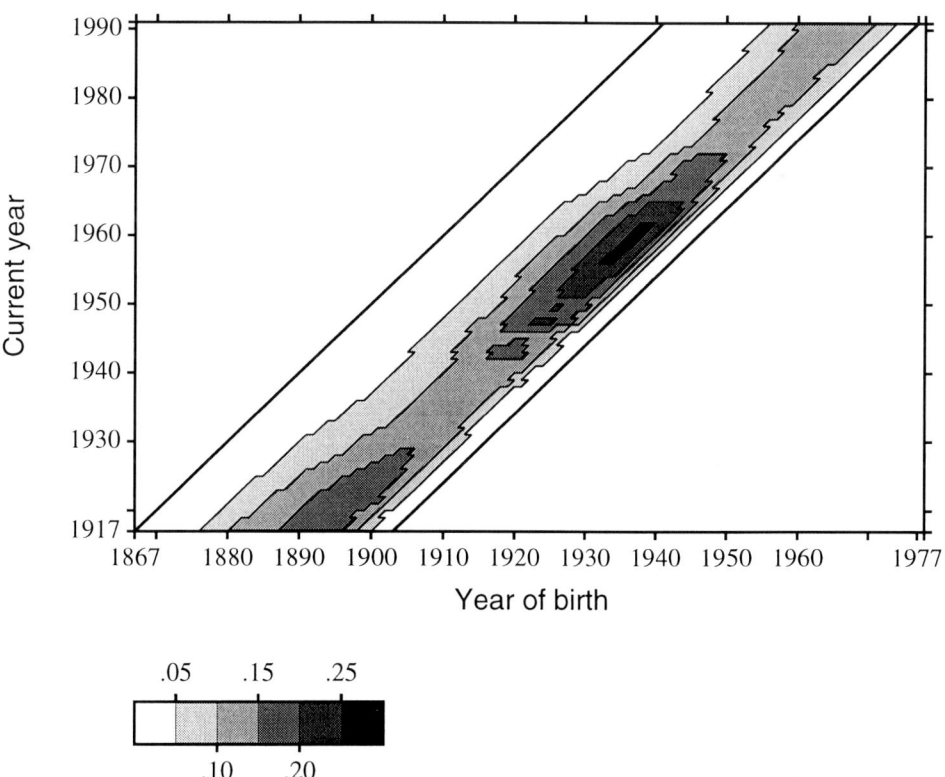

**Figure 7.** US birth rates by current year and year of birth, with selected contour lines from 0.05 to 0.25, and from current year 1917 to 1990 and year of birth 1867 to 1977.

The fertility data pertaining to earlier years, especially the years before 1950, have to be interpreted with caution since they are reconstructions based on interviews taken in 1982. The general pattern seems reassuringly plausible: over the course of the 1940s and 1950s birth rates were fairly stable, with some tendency toward increase. This is consistent with trends in improvements in living standards, and the absence of widespread contraception, during this period.

Figure 9 shows the fluctuating pattern of Finnish fertility since 1776; it is based on data supplied by Wolfgang Lutz. The various wars and famines that disrupted life in Finland are apparent on the map, as is the substantial decline in fertility after World War I, especially at older ages. Lutz also notes the decline in fertility apparent in the eighteenth century: this represents the culmination of a nuptiality transition starting about 1750.

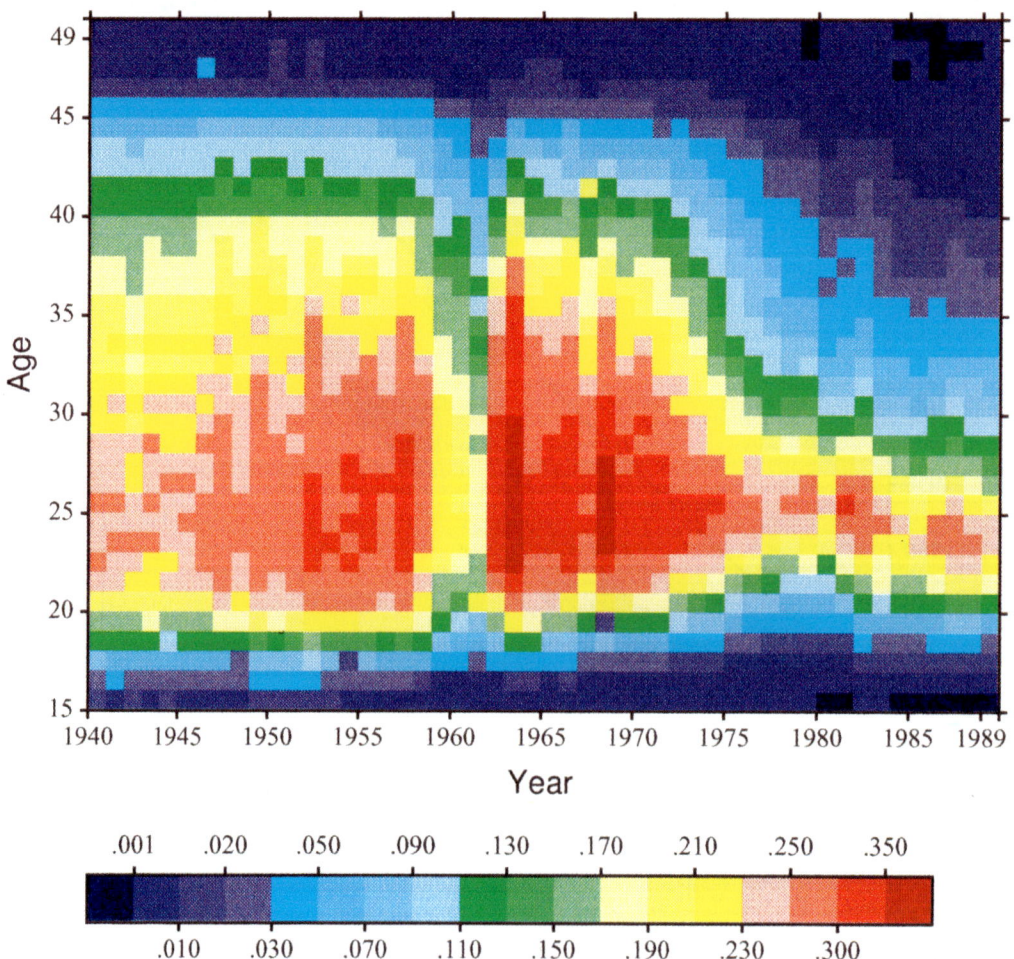

**Figure 8.** Chinese birth rates, with contours selectively placed from 0.001 to 0.35 and from age 15 to 49 and year 1940 to 1989.

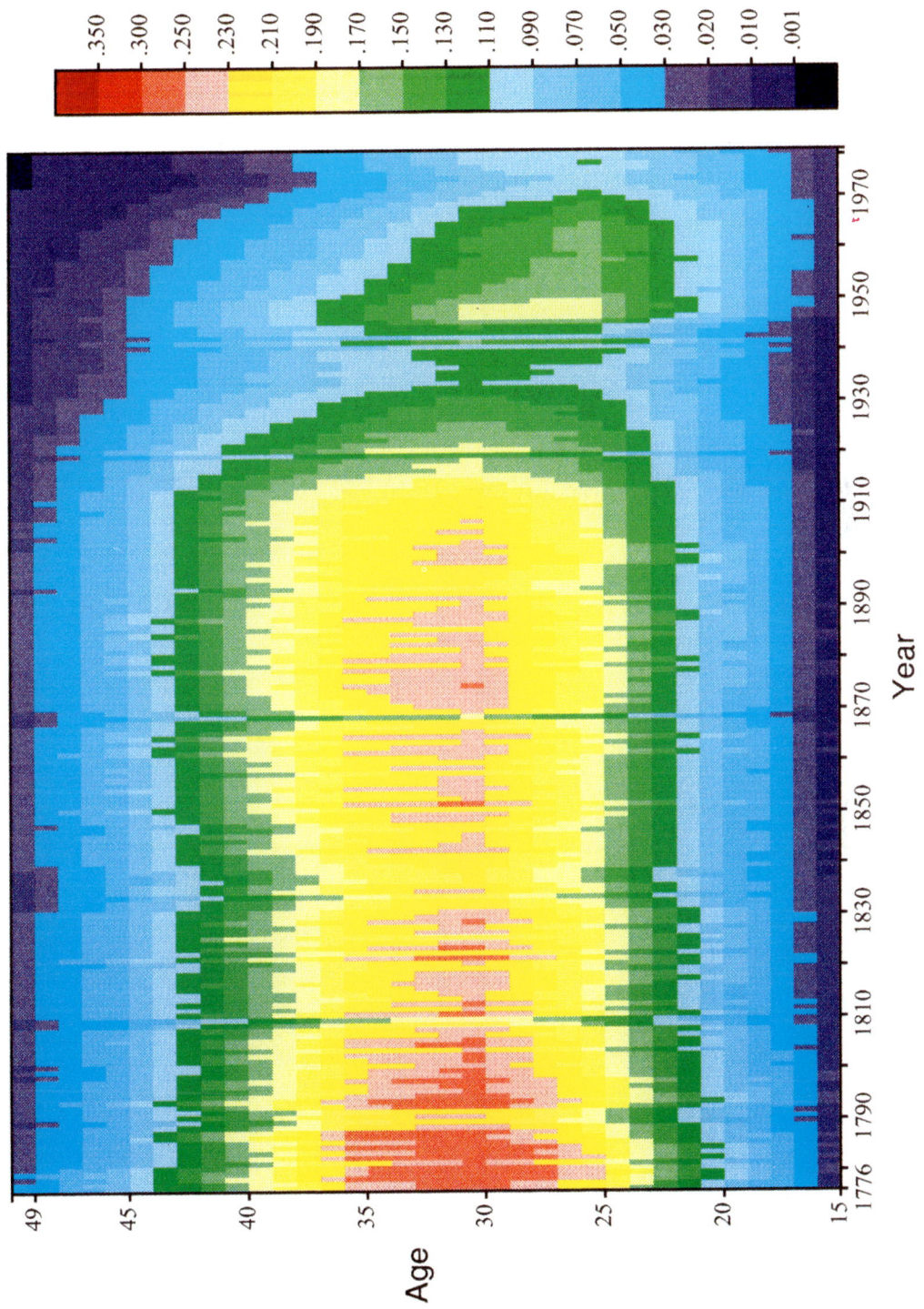

**Figure 9.** Finnish birth rates, with contours selectively placed from 0.001 to 0.35, and from age 15 to 49 and year 1776 to 1970.

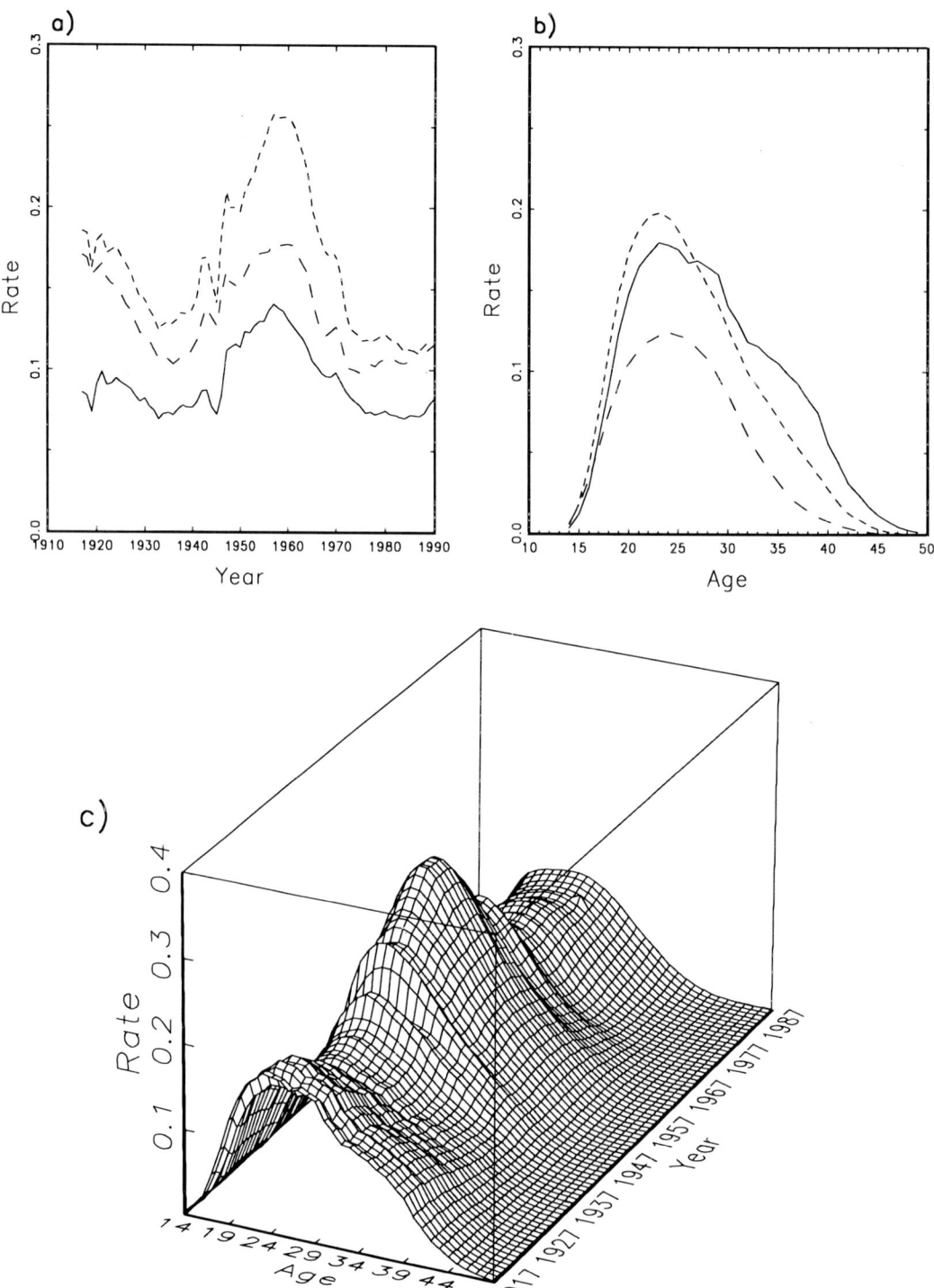

**Figure 10.** (a) US birth rates from year 1917 to 1990 at ages 18 (solid line), 23 (small dashes), and 28 (large dashes); (b) US birth rates from age 14 to 49 in 1920 (solid line), 1950 (small dashes), and 1980 (large dashes); (c) Three-dimensional plot of US birth rates from age 14 to 49 and year 1917 to 1990.

# 8. Alternative graphic displays of U.S. female fertility

The most commonly used method for displaying demographic rates over age and time is to plot the rates over time for selected ages or over age for selected times. In Figure 10(a), for instance, U.S. birth rates are plotted over time at ages 18, 23, and 28 and in Figure 10(b) the birth rates are plotted from age 14 to 49 for years 1920, 1950, and 1980. Comparison of Figures 10(a) and 10(b) with the Lexis maps presented in Figures 5, 6, and 7 reveals some of the strengths and weaknesses of these alternative graphic displays. The Lexis maps present far more information and give an overview of the entire surface. The plots over age and time focus attention on trends and fluctuations in those two directions. The Lexis maps might be compared to a lavish Chinese banquet, whereas the graphs over age and time are more like a delicate Japanese dinner.

Figures 10(c) and 11 show plots of the US birth rate data drawn from a three-dimensional perspective. With appropriate software, it is possible not only to produce but also to rotate such three-dimensional pictures on a computer monitor so that they can be viewed from various angles: the three perspectives shown in Figure 11 suggest how informative this kind of rotation can be. Clearly, three-dimensional plots are an important tool for demographers.

A three-dimensional plot sacrifices some of the richness of detail that is clearly portrayed on the corresponding contour map; furthermore, it is difficult on a three-dimensional plot to relate a point on the surface to the exact age and year underlying the point. Just as architects, surveyors, and engineers rely on contour maps for site planning and cartographers use contour and topographical maps in depicting a variety of terrains and surfaces, demographers will also undoubtedly find that for some purposes contour maps are the most appropriate means for representing a population surface. Fisher's (1982) comprehensive comparison of an array of different methods for "mapping information" reveals the relative advantages, for many purposes, of "the combined use of contour lines and tones".

Any graphical method has its strengths and weaknesses. Our point is simply that demographers should consider adding contour maps to their toolkit, to supplement graphs of rates over age and time, three-dimensional plots, age pyramids, and other techniques.

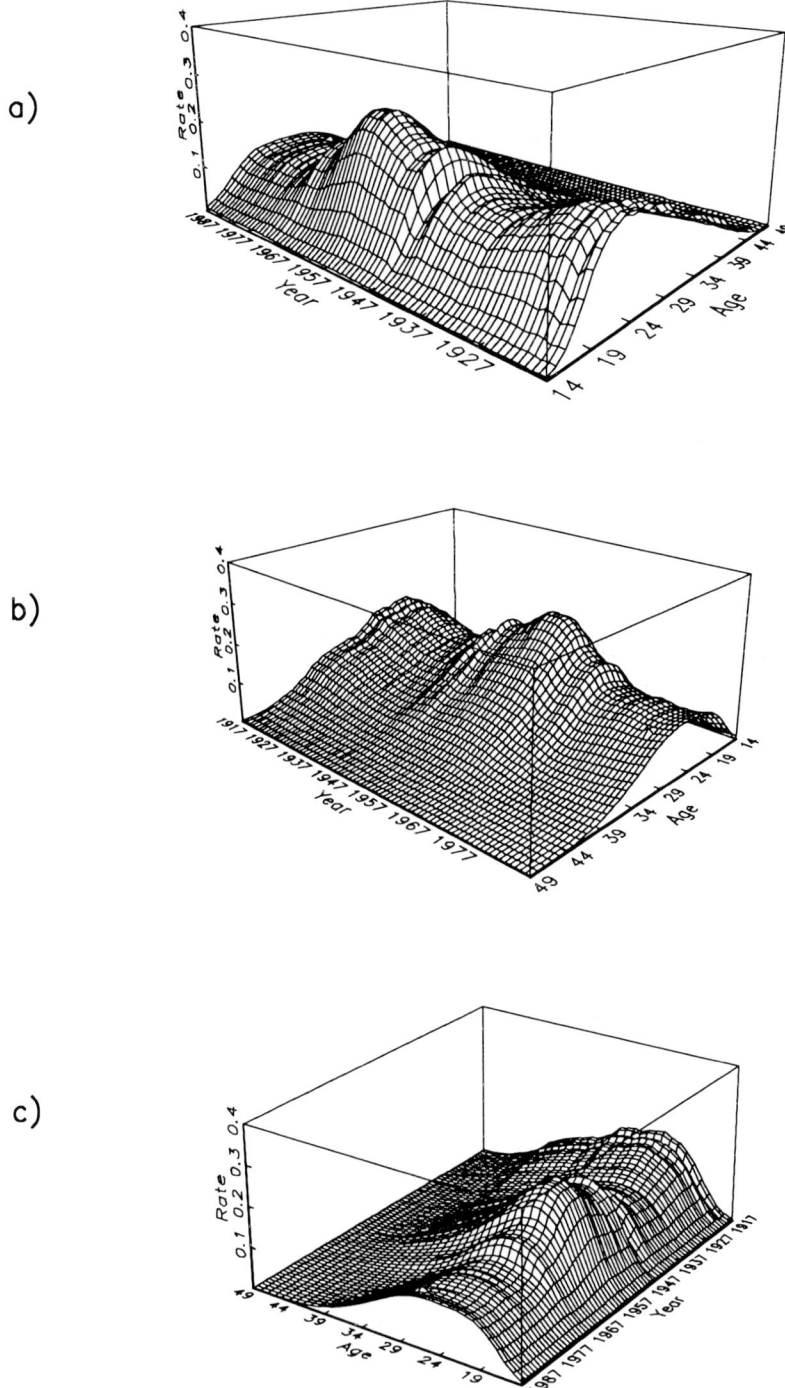

**Figure 11.** Three-dimensional plots of US birth rates.

# 9. The female populations of Sweden and Japan at older ages

Surfaces of population levels are especially important in the theory of population dynamics, as discussed by Arthur and Vaupel (1984). Figure 12(a) presents such a surface, of Swedish female population levels from age 0 to age 111 from years 1861 to 1993, on data compiled by Lundström (Vaupel and Lundström 1994) and Wilmoth. For each year of age and time, the map displays the estimated population on July 1. The patterns reflect differences in cohort sizes, the impact of mortality, and the effects, especially before age 50 and year 1920, of out-migration. The strong diagonals reveal

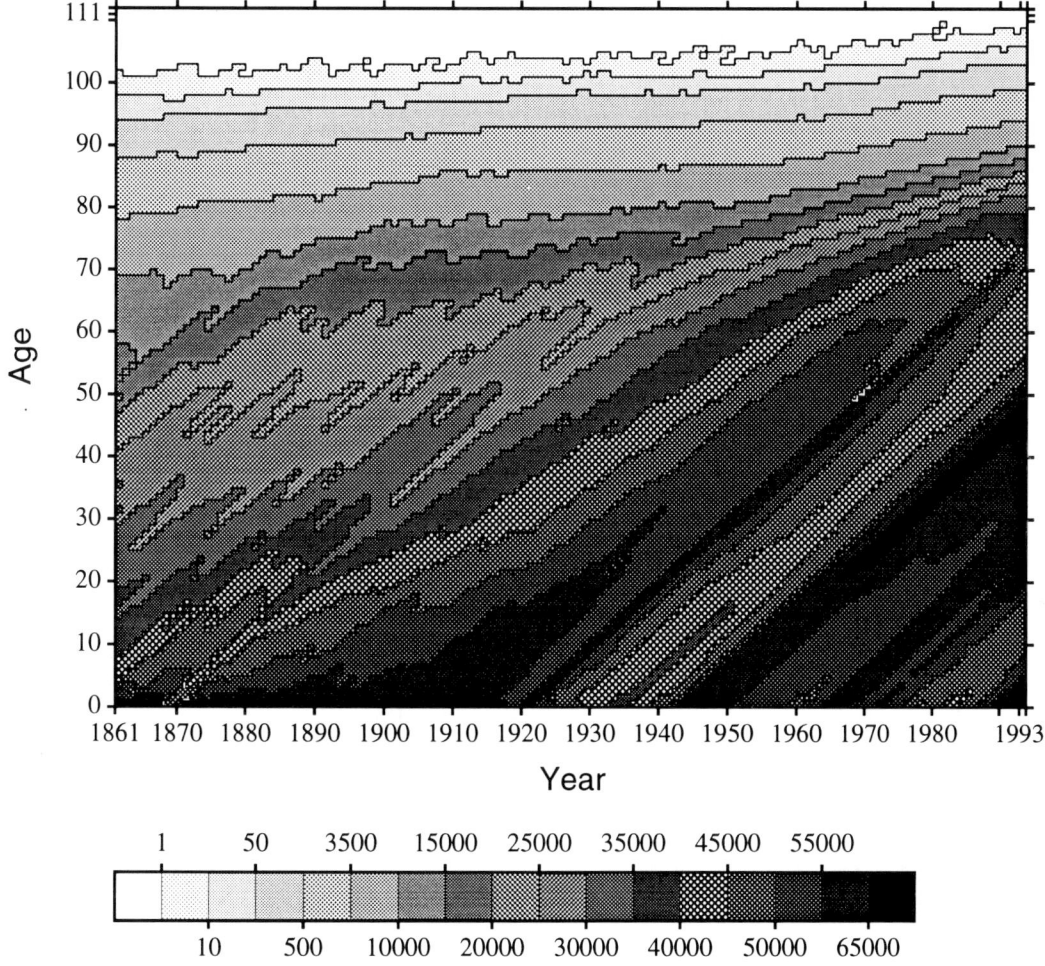

**Figure 12(a).** Swedish female population, with contour lines from 1 to 65000, and from age 0 to 111 and year 1861 to 1993.

variations in surviving populations in adjacent cohorts. The surface falls off sharply with age, as death takes its toll. In addition, the surface rises substantially with time. The increase in the number of the elderly is partly due to an increase in the size of birth cohorts, but improved survival, especially at advanced ages, plays the major role (Vaupel and Jeune, 1995).

To depict the change that has occurred over time in age-specific population levels, or such other demographic statistics as fertility or mortality rates, it is useful to draw Lexis maps of relative surfaces on which the value of the statistic at each point is calculated relative to the value of the statistic in some base year. Figure 12(b), for example, presents Swedish female population levels relative to the average level in 1861-1870. Thus, the figure dramatically displays the explosion of the population of the oldest-

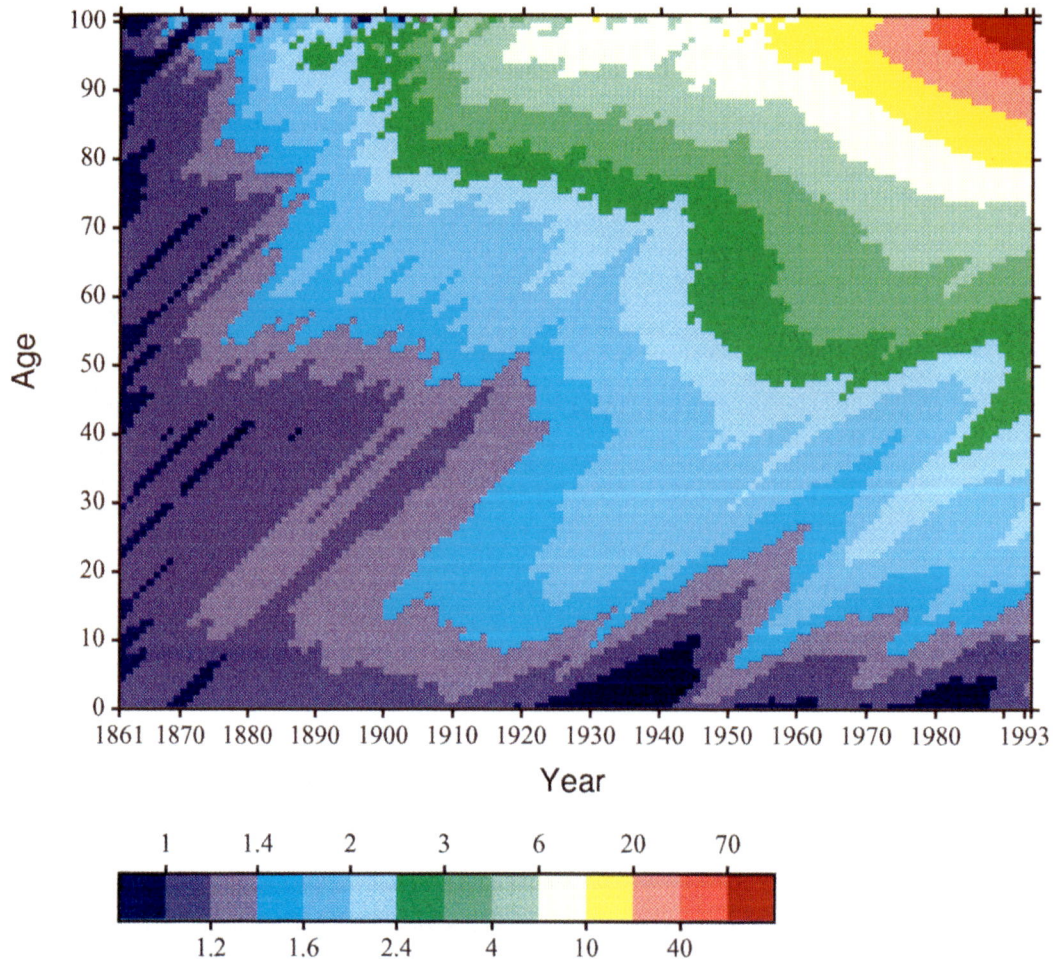

**Figure 12(b).** Swedish female population relative to average level in 1861-1870, from 0 to 100 and year 1861 to 1993, with contours selectively from 1 to 70.

old. Whereas the number of 50-year-olds rose three or four fold from the 1860s to the 1980s, the number of centenarians increased by more than 70-fold.

Figure 13 reveals the order-of-magnitude increases in the numbers of female octogenarians, nonagenarians, and centenarians in Japan since 1950; the figure is based on data supplied by John Wilmoth. The white triange in the northwest corner of the map is terra incognita: no data were available for these ages and years. The largely white area to the right of the frontier of knowledge depicts the ages and years at which there were no survivors. The long light-grey diagonals at the top of the map may follow the exceptional longevity of the last members of some birth cohorts; alternatively, they may be traces of errors in the statistics.

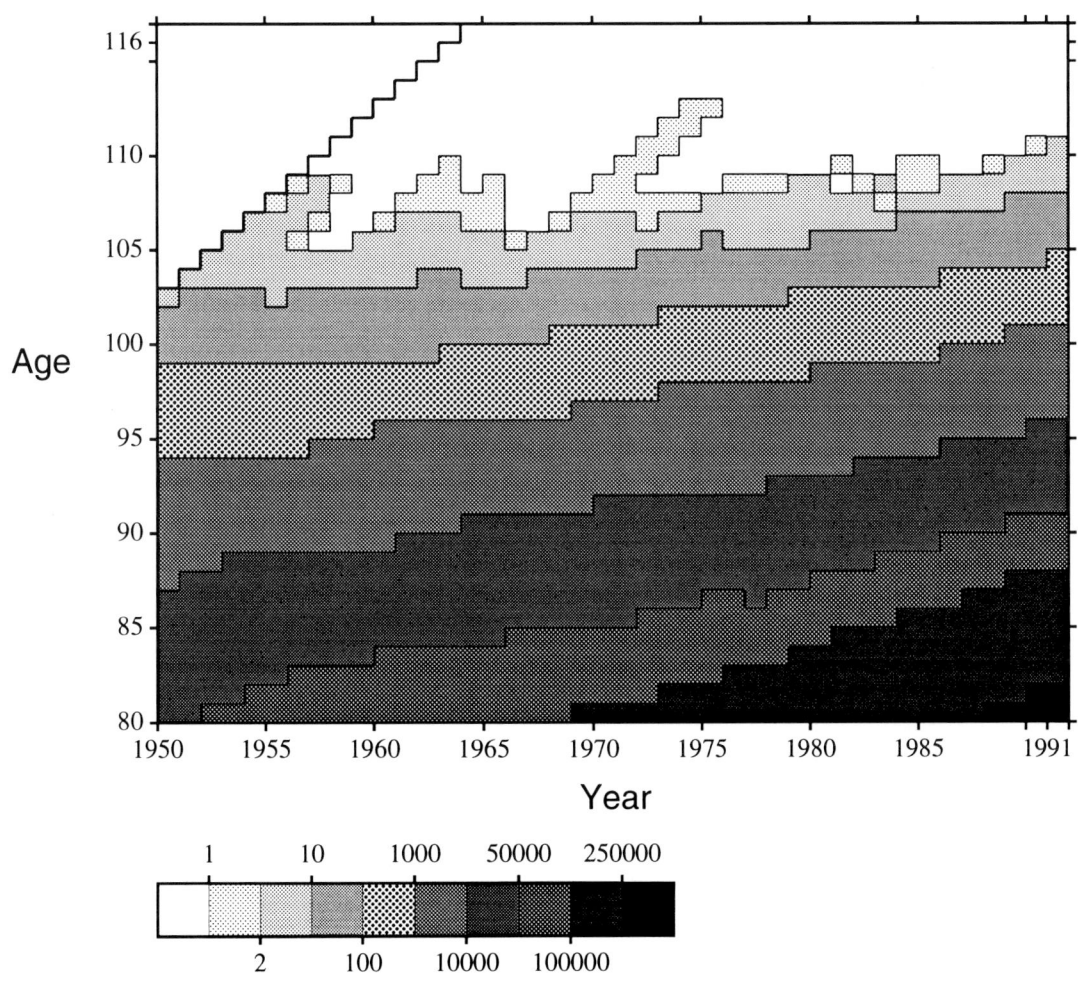

**Figure 13.** Japanese female population, with contour lines from 1 to 250000, and from age 80 to 116 and year 1950 to 1991.

# 10. Relative surfaces of Italian mortality, US fertility, and Belgian population

Two applications of relative contour maps are shown in Figures 14 and 15. Figure 14 displays age-specific probabilities of death for Italian males relative to their levels in 1925, a year roughly halfway through the period studied. The map clearly reveals the great progress that has been made in reducing mortality at the youngest ages compared with the slow progress at the oldest ages. The map also puts the devastation of World War I into perspective: World War I essentially erased a half century of progress, but the setback was temporary and pre-World War I mortality rates at most ages were achieved and surpassed within a decade or so.

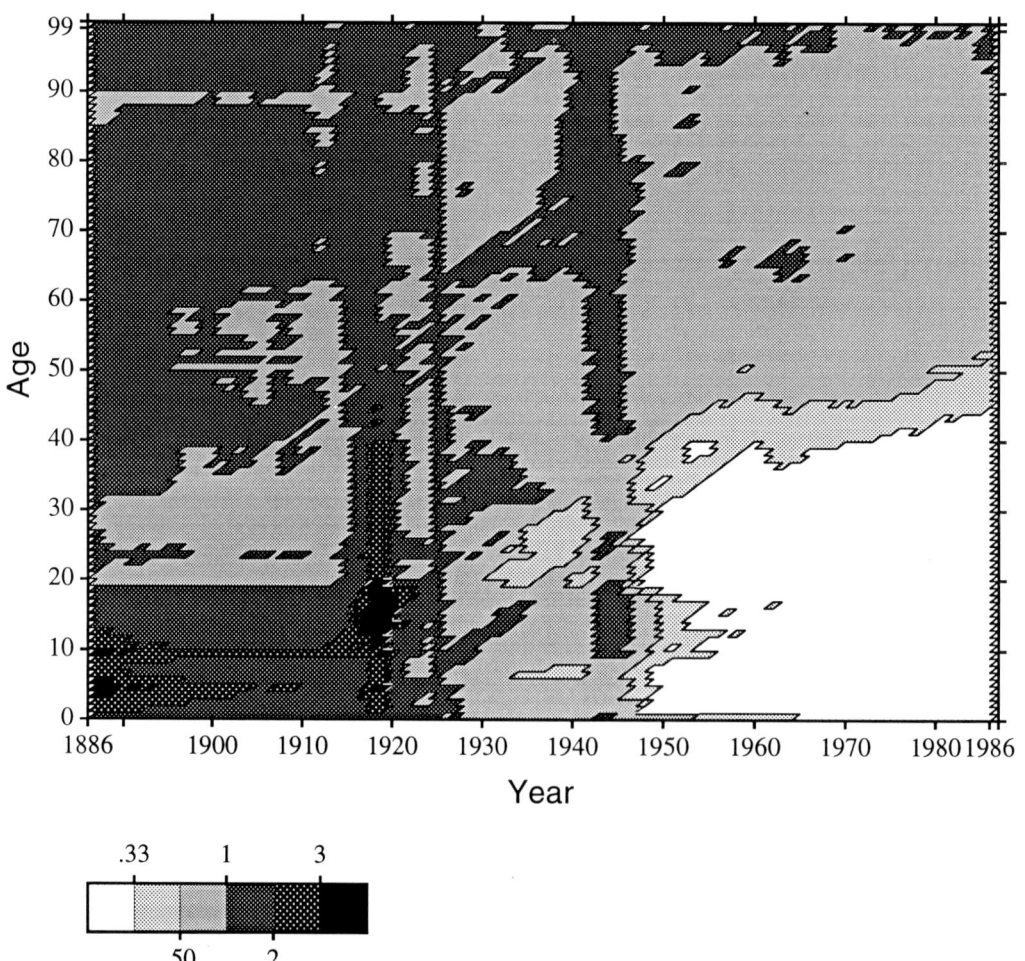

**Figure 14.** Probabilities of death for Italian males relative to age-specific 1925 levels, with contour lines from 0.33 to 3, from age 0 to 99 and year 1886 to 1986.

Figure 15 presents age-specific birth rates for US females relative to their level in 1980. The map highlights the dramatic reduction before 1980 in birth rates above age 35, compared with the less radical (relative) changes at younger ages. Even the baby boom pales in significance when viewed from this perspective. The map also highlights the increase in fertility after 1980, especially at older ages.

Instead of dividing a demographic array by the age-specific statistics for a particular year the array could be divided by the period-specific statistics for a particular age. For example, Figure 16 shows probabilities of death for Italian males at various ages relative to infant mortality in the appropriate year. The map is smoothed, with averages being taken over 5 x 5 squares of age and time: this smoothing reduces mortality at age 0. The falling contours on the top half of the map emphasize a trend that was less apparent in Figure 1(b), namely that progress against mortality at older ages has been slower than that at younger ages. In 1886, death rates at age 80 were less than the level

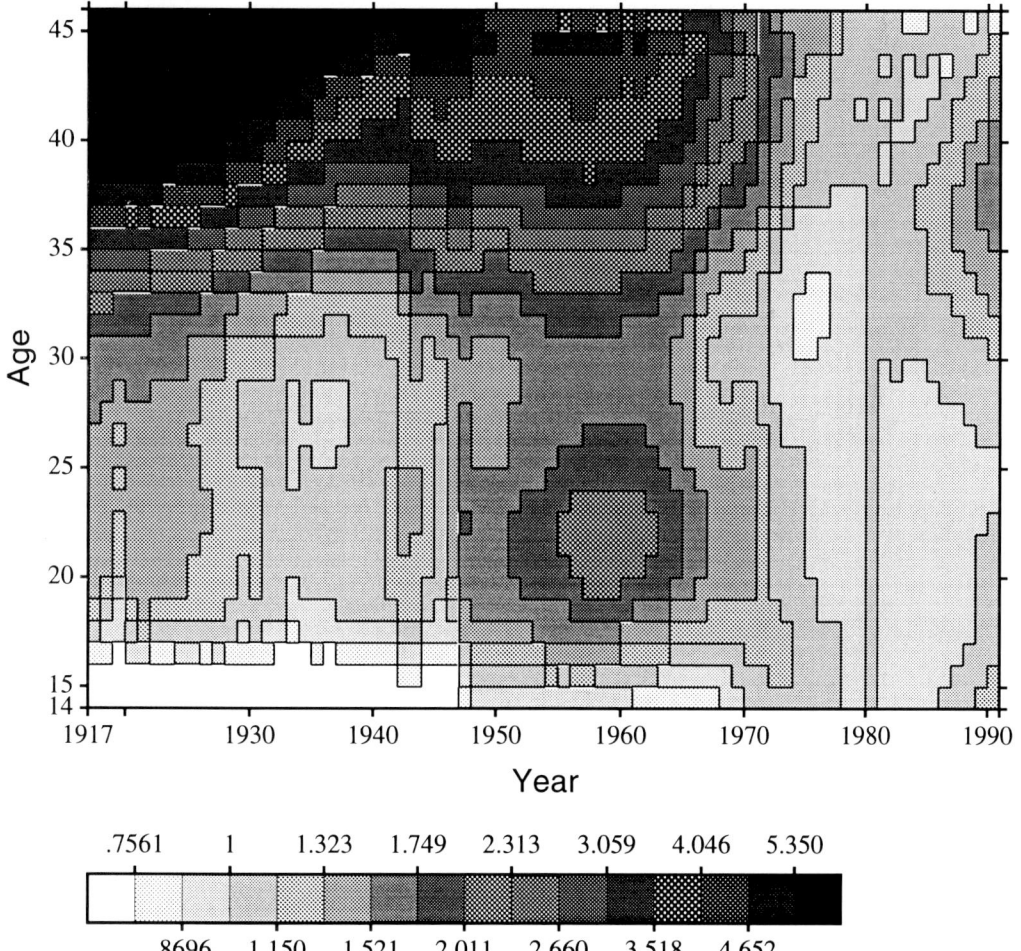

**Figure 15.** US birth rates relative to age-specific 1980 levels, with contour lines from 0.7561 to 5.350 at multiples of 1.15, from age 14 to 45 and year 1917 to 1990.

of infant mortality; a century later, death rates at age 80 were more than 6 times higher than the prevailing infant rates.

Demographic statistics can also be expressed relative to some composite age-specific or period-specific measure. Figures 17 and 18 provide two examples. To produce Figure 17, Belgian age-specific female population levels (from Veys, 1983) were divided by the total Belgian female population in each year. Thus the map gives contours of the age distribution of the population, i.e., the percentage of the population in each year that are at various ages. The diagonal traces of the small cohorts born during World Wars I and II are apparent, as is the general trend of the age composition of the population to shift upward to older ages. As a proportion of the population, 70-year-olds were as important in 1970 as 40-year-olds were in 1892.

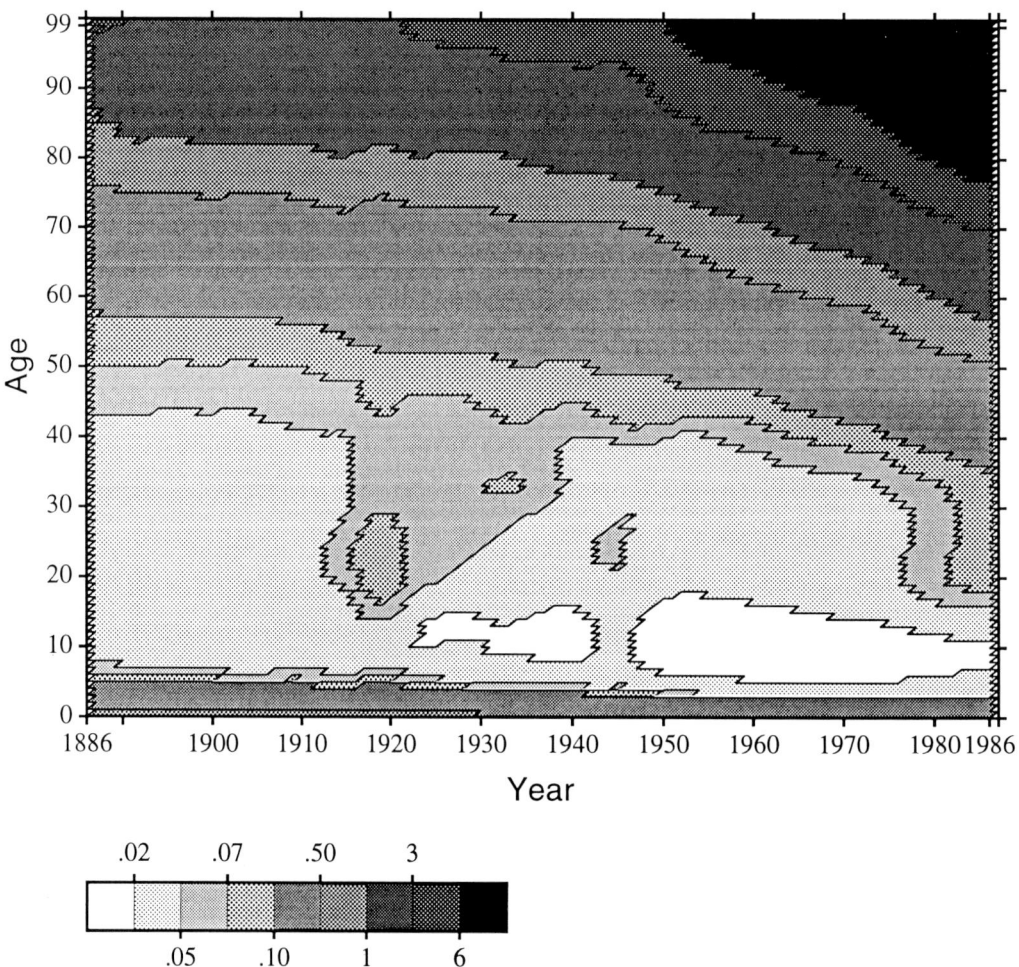

**Figure 16.** Probabilities of death for Italian males relative to infant mortality, with contour lines from 0.02 to 6.0, smoothed on a 5 x 5 square, and from age 0 to 99 and year 1886 to 1986.

Figure 18, which is based on US fertility data, is similar in nature except that the contours pertain to cumulative levels up through age 49 relative to the total level over all ages. The map can be interpreted as showing the proportion of all births in a given year that occurred to women of some age or less - in a synthetic population in which there were equal numbers of women at each age. The general trend is downward, especially at older ages: a greater cumulative proportion of children is being born each year to younger women. This trend runs through the periods of baby boom and bust, but there is some reversal of the trend between ages 25 and 35 after 1980.

Finally, it may sometimes be useful to examine Lexis maps based on statistics relative to a cohort-specific measure rather than either an age-specific or period-specific measure. Consider, for instance, Figure 19, which is similar to Figure 18 except that

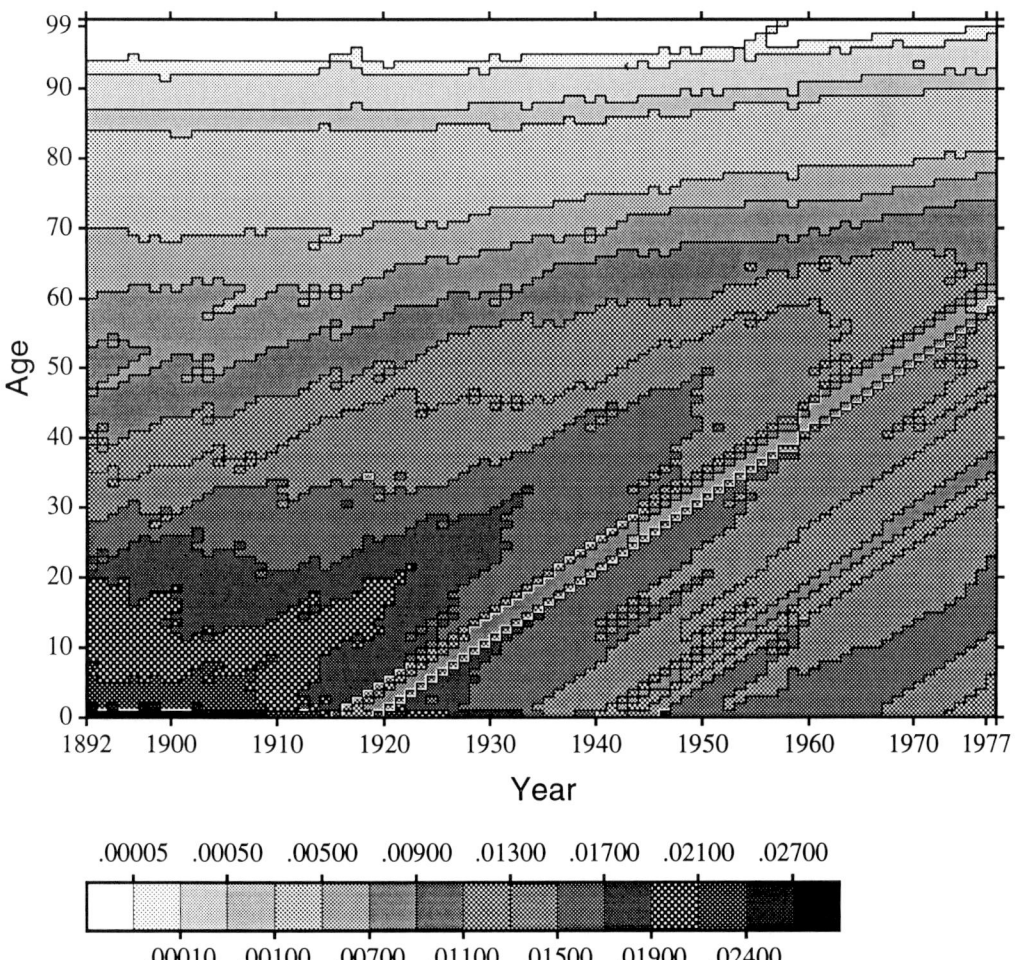

**Figure 17.** Age-distribution of Belgian female population, with contour lines selectively placed from 0.00005 to 0.027, and from age 0 to 99 and year 1892 to 1977.

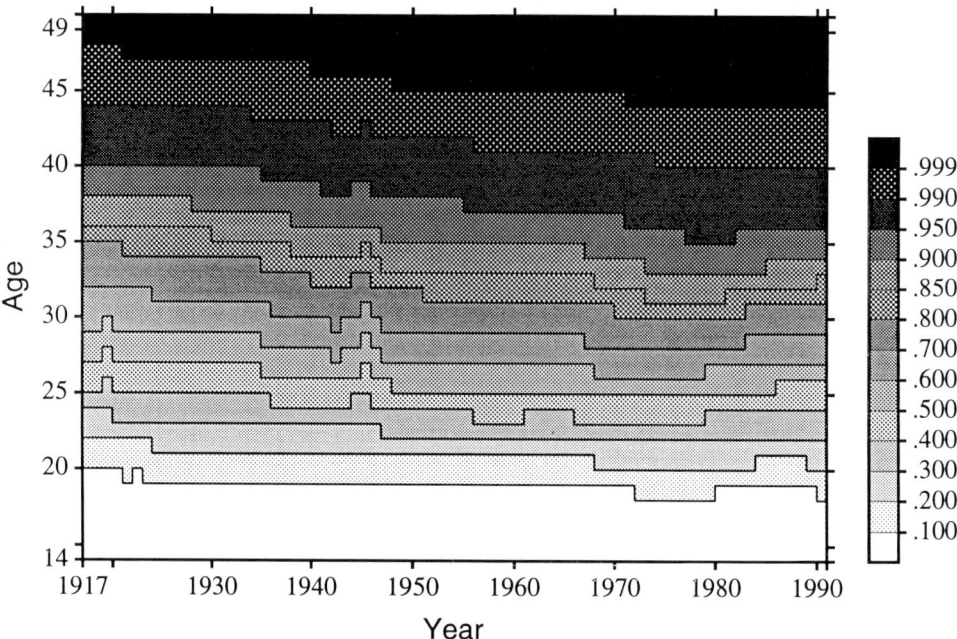

**Figure 18.** Cumulative distribution of US births by age and year, with contour lines selectively placed from 0.1 to 0.999, and from age 14 to 49 and year 1917 to 1990.

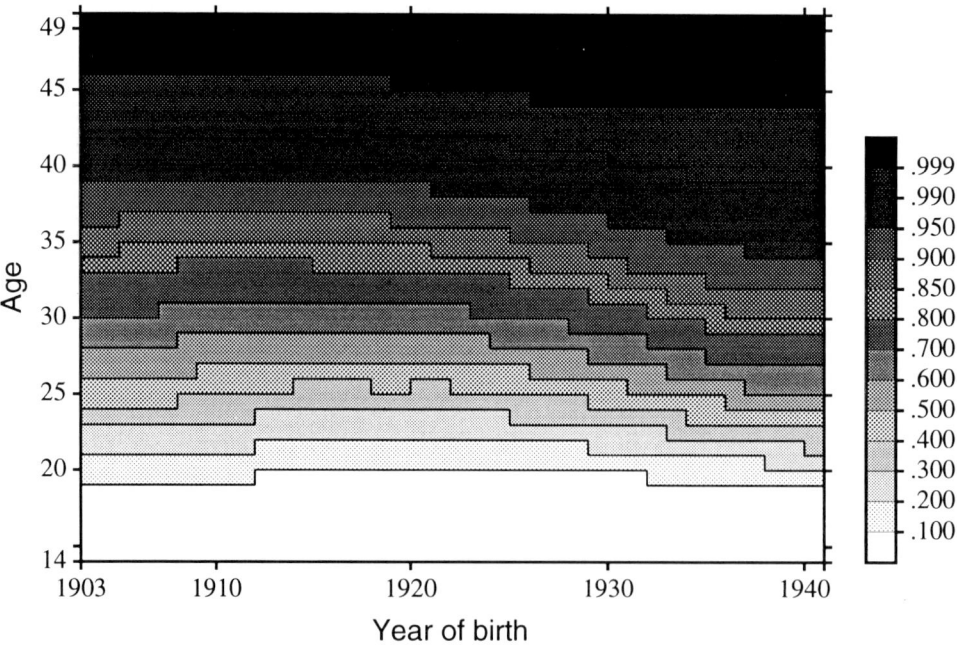

**Figure 19.** Cumulative distribution of US births by age and year of birth of mother, with contour lines selectively placed from 0.1 to 0.999, and from age 14 to 49 and year of birth 1903 to 1940.

cumulative fertility is computed relative to total cohort fertility up through age 49. The general trend is up, then down. Consider, for instance, the .5 contour line. For the 1903 birth cohort, this contour line indicates that half of the children were born by age 26. For the cohorts born around 1915, half the children were born by age 27, whereas for the cohorts born in 1940, half the children were born by age 24.

# 11. Small multiples

To compare global patterns among several population surfaces it may be useful to shrink contour maps and present several of them on the same page: Tufte (1983) calls this the "small multiples" approach. Figure 20 presents maps of US birth rates at various parities: in Figure 20(a), first birth rates (i.e., the proportion of all women of some age in some year who have their first child) are displayed; in Figure 20(b), second birth rates are displayed, and so on. In each of the small multiples, the same contour levels are used. Because the birth rates shown in these figures are all based on the same denominator at any particular age and time, namely, the total number of women of that age in that year, the maps can in effect be added together to approximate the total birth rate at any age and time; the result is approximate because seventh and higher birth orders are omitted. In other words, the maps decompose total fertility into the contribution made at different parities.

This decomposition indicates that the absolute fluctuations in numbers of first and second children were more significant, in creating the waves of baby booms and busts, than the absolute fluctuations in higher-order births: for both first and second children, fertility rates at the peak age (around 20 for first births and 22 for second births) were about 5% points higher around 1960 than they were around 1935, whereas for fourth and higher birth orders, the absolute difference was only 1-2%. As shown in Figure 5, the absolute difference between the total fertility rate at age 22 between 1935 and 1960 was about 14%, so that the change in first and second birth rates accounted for roughly two-thirds of the total change.

One aspect of the recent baby boom that is strikingly revealed by the maps in Figure 20 is that the peak of the boom occurred around 1960 at all six parities, at ages that drift upward from about 20 in the case of first births to about 30 in the case of sixth births. The maps also show the trend in the 1970s toward greater first and second birth

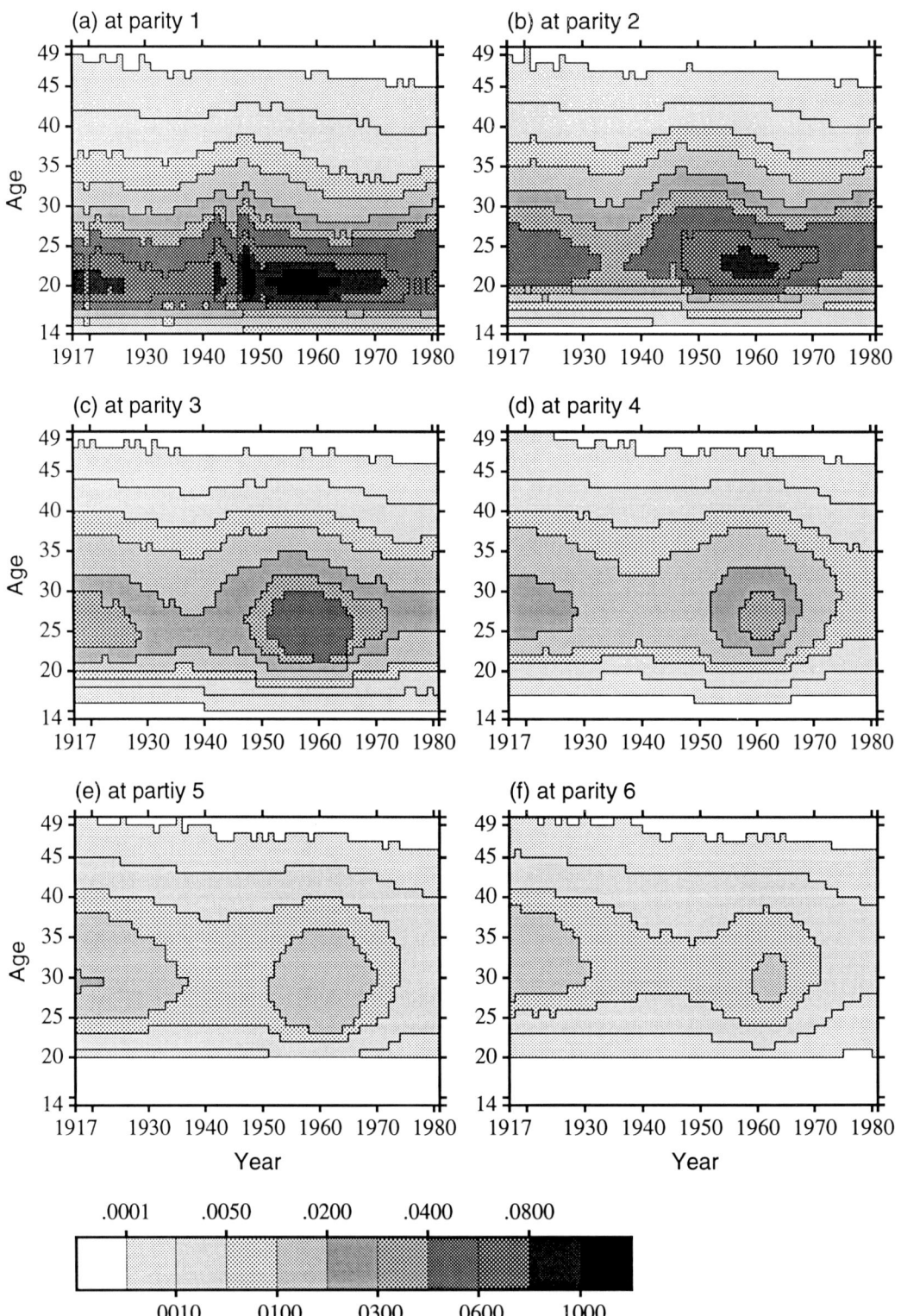

**Figure 20.** US birth rates with contour lines selectively placed from 0.0001 to 0.1 and from age 14 to 49 and year 1917 to 1980.

rates among women in their late 20s and in their 30s, although fourth and higher-order birth rates for these women (as well as women at other ages) continued to decline. In general, the maps provide further evidence of the importance of age and period effects but substantial cohort effects are less apparent. It might be noted, however, that the sharp increase in first births started in the late 1940s among women around age 20, whereas the increase in sixth births occured around 1960 for women around age 30.

The six small multiples shown in Figure 20 are included on the computer diskette we have produced, together with a program that displays the maps in sequence, either slowly or quickly, as a kind of demographic movie. The movie is not only visually striking, but also informative. In particular, movement in the cohort direction is apparent, as it should be since a woman cannot have her third child until after she has had her second child.

Figure 21 presents another illustration of the use of small multiples, this time to compare mortality from ages 15 to 49 for years 1910 to 1965 for Italian, French, and Belgian males and females. The effects of World Wars I and II are most prominent in this period and for these ages; the maps graphically depict the different impact of the two wars among the two sexes in the three countries. The diagonal swatch of high mortality for Italian males [Figure 21(a)] born around the turn of the century, discussed earlier, does not show up on any of the other maps in Figure 21. The prevalence of many small blocks on the Belgian maps [Figure 21(c) and 21(d)] indicates some scattered noise or local fluctuations, perhaps attributable to the smaller size of the Belgian population compared with that of Italy or France or to irregularities in the available mortality data.

Figure 22 displays relative mortality for males and females in England and Wales, Sweden, and Italy from age 5 to 79 for years 1870 to 1978. In each case, the probability of death for a given age is relative to the probability at that age in 1870. Thus, the maps provide a picture of the pattern of progress made in reducing mortality since 1870. They are analogous to the tables with rough contour lines in Kermack et al. (1934); Preston and van der Walle (1978) and Coale and Kisker (1985) present similar tables. These analysts ascribe the diagonal contours in their tables to cohort effects.

The maps in Figure 22 provide a richer, more detailed picture of the various local and global patterns in the changes in mortality, in vertical, horizontal, and diagonal directions. Some diagonal trends are evident, especially for females in England and Wales [Figure 21(f)], but it is also evident that age and period effects play a substantial role in the evolution of mortality. The light rectangles in the lower right corners of all six maps show the rapid progress in reducing mortality at younger ages since World War II; the darkness of the remaining three quadrants of the maps displays the slower rate of

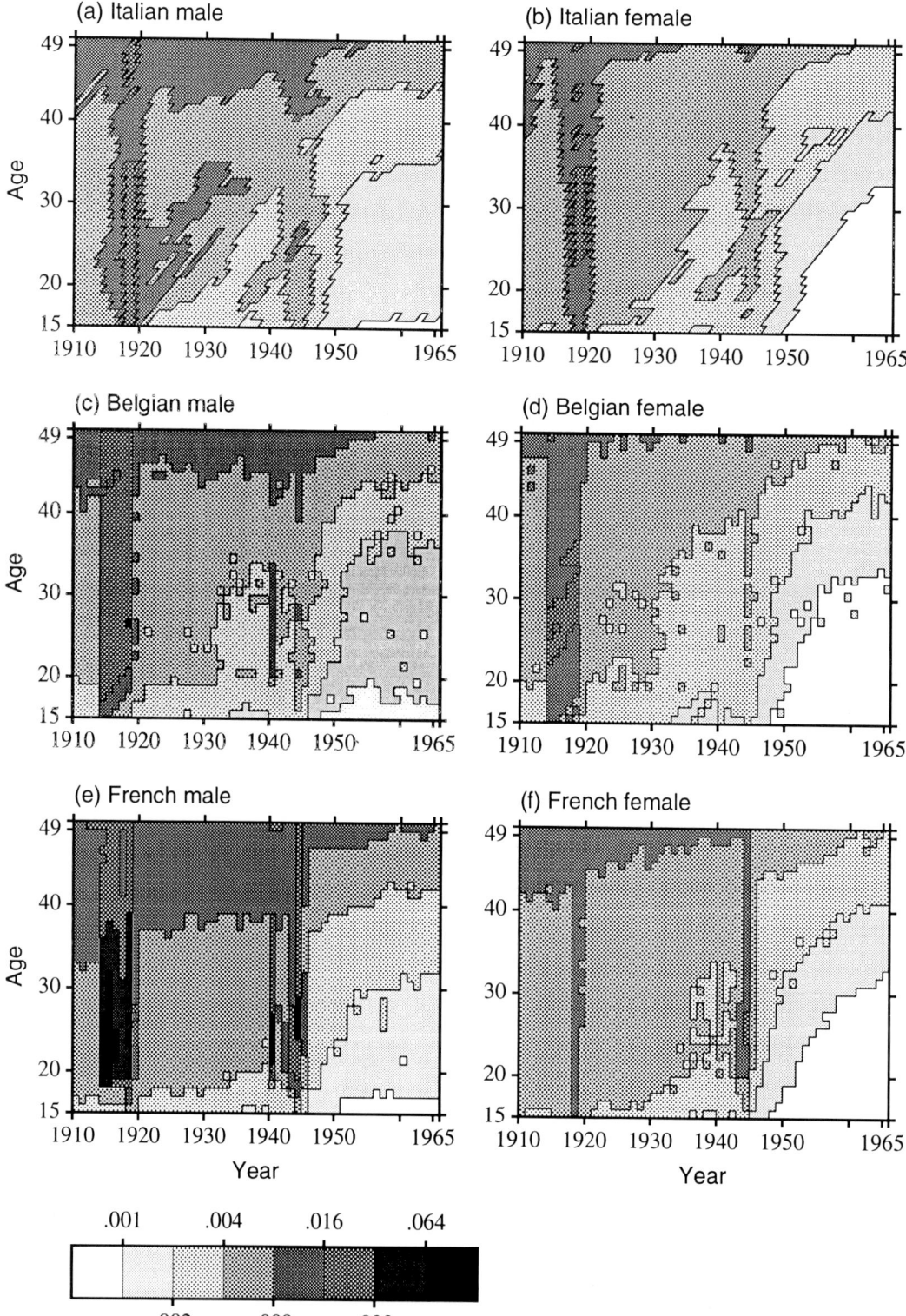

**Figure 21.** Probabilities of death for males and females in Italy, Belgium, and France, with contour lines from 0.001 to 0.064 at multiples of 2, and from age 15 to 49 and year 1910 to 1965.

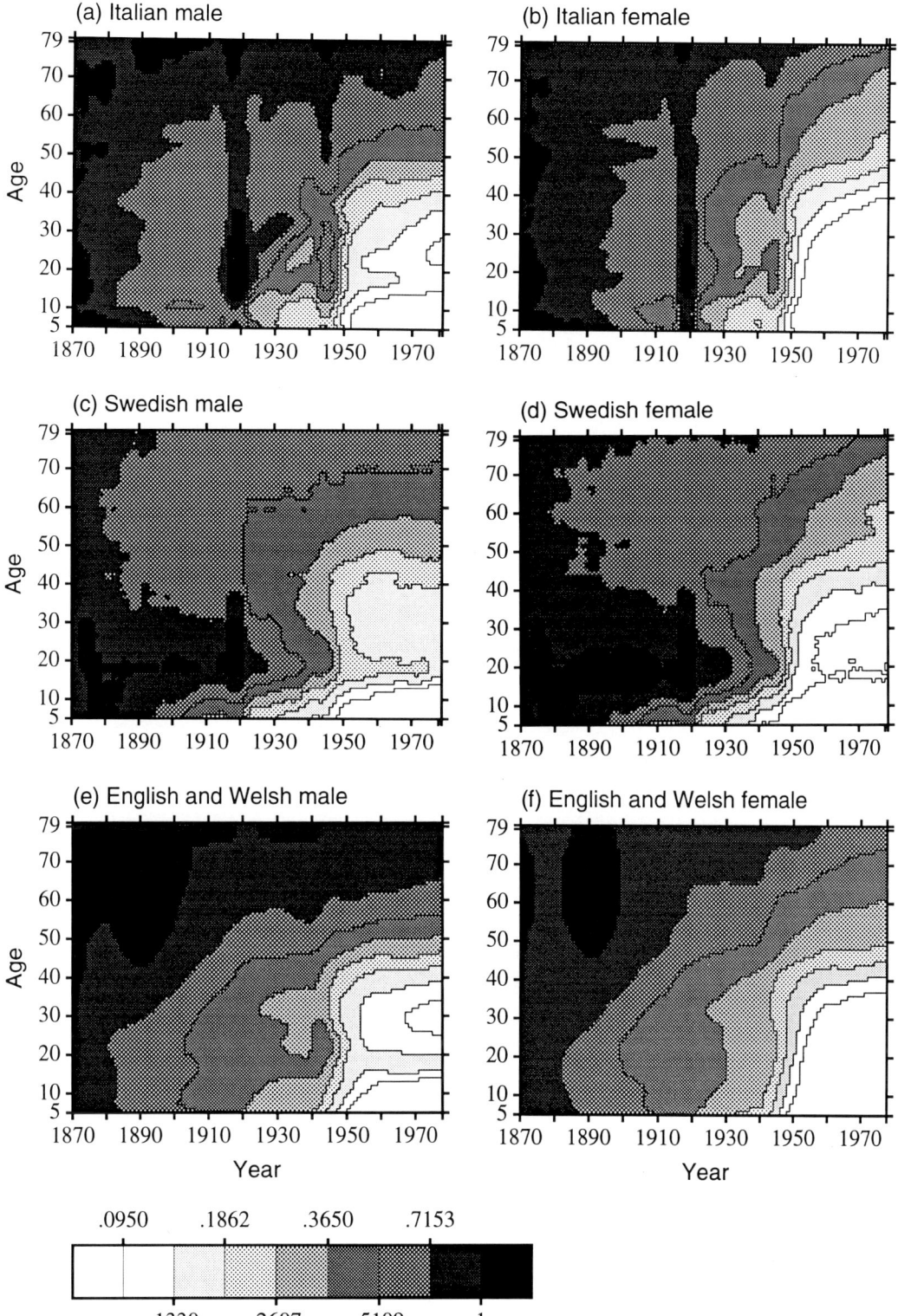

**Figure 22.** Probabilities of death relative to 1870 age-specific levels for males and females in Italy, Sweden, and England and Wales, with contour lines from 0.095 to 1.0 at multiples of 1.4, smoothed on a square, and from age 5 to 79 and year 1870 to 1978.

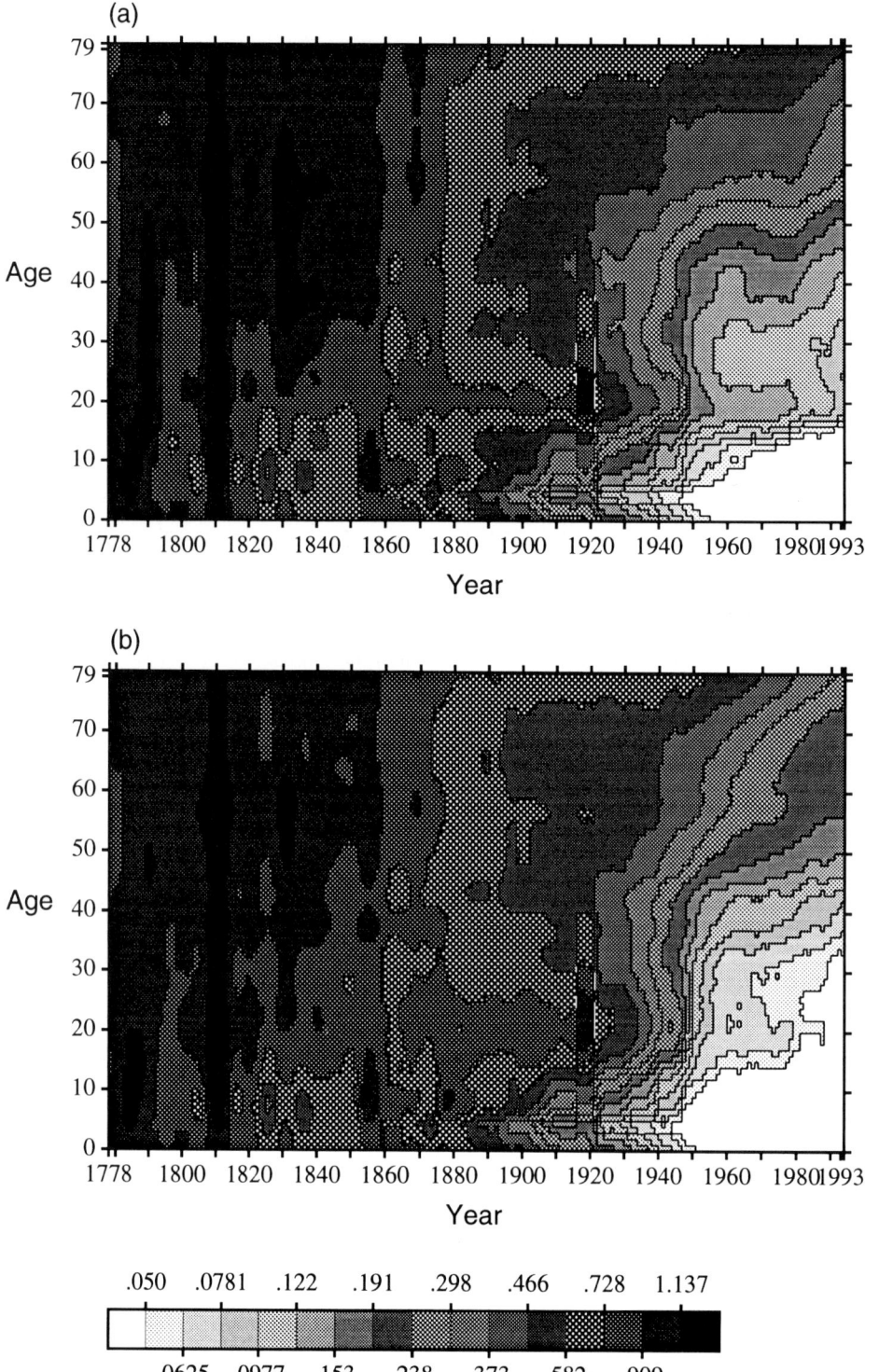

**Figure 23.** Probabilities of death in Sweden relative to age-specific levels from 1778 to 1799, with contour lines from 0.05 to 1.137 at multiples of 1.15, smoothed on a 5 x 5 square, and from age 0 to 79 and year 1778 to 1993: (a) male; (b) female.

progress at older ages and during earlier years. Note that the light rectangles in the lower right corners are divided, for males but not for females, by a darker stripe, indicating relatively slow progress against mortality at, roughly, ages 16 to 20.

The maps in Figure 22 for the three countries were produced using different kinds of data. As noted earlier, death rates for Italy were available for single years of time and age. For Sweden, the rates were generally available for five-year periods; before 1880 the rates were for five-year age categories and afterward for single years of age. Finally, for England and Wales, the rates were available for five-year age categories for single years of time about once per decade. Differences in the smoothness of the maps, especially for England and Wales compared with Italy, are probably largely attributable to these differences in data richness.

In the analyses of Kermack et al. (1934), Preston and van der Walle (1978), and Coale and Kisker (1990), death rates were taken relative to a period earlier than 1870, the underlying assumption being that at an early enough period there would have been no systematic pattern of progress against mortality. Figure 23 shows probabilities of death for Swedish males (a) and females (b) relative to the average levels at each age in the period from 1778 to 1799. The figure reveals the fluctuating pattern of mortality before the middle of the nineteenth century and the general pattern of progress against mortality subsequently. The pattern is clearly more complex than a pure cohort-effect model would suggest.

A direct way of considering the hypothesis that "a cohort carries its mortality level with it" is to examine mortality surfaces that are calculated relative to a cohort's mortality levels. In Figure 24, for instance, in each of the six surfaces shown the probability of death at each age and year was divided by the probability at that age for the cohort born in 1870. The patterns that emerge show some strong diagonals, but it is apparent that there are also important effects in horizontal and vertical directions. Interpretation of these and similar surfaces should also be tempered by the realization that diagonal patterns can emerge not only as a result of cohort effects but also as the result of the interaction of period and age effects.

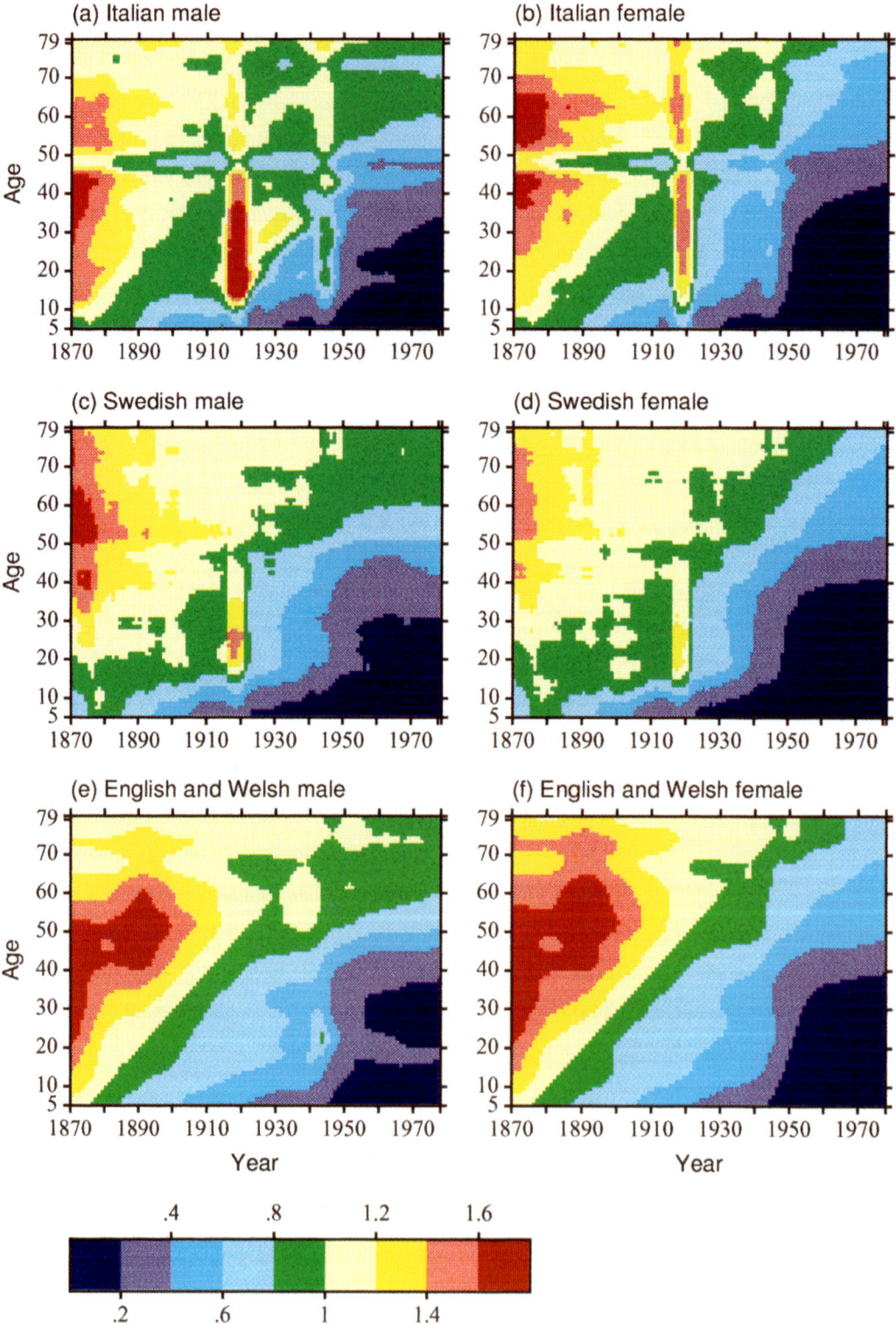

**Figure 24.** Probabilities of death relative to 1870 age-specific cohort levels (in color), with contours selectively placed from 0.2 to 1.6, smoothed on a 5 x 5 square, and from age 5 to 79 and year 1870 to 1978 for Italy and Sweden and year 1870 to 1977 for England and Wales.

# 12. Ratio surfaces

Instead of using small multiples or computer movies, another approach to comparing two or more demographic surfaces is to compute some new surfaces that represent at every point either the difference or the ratio of the height of one of the original surfaces to another. Figure 25(a), for instance, shows the ratio of female to male probabilities of death in Italy, smoothed on a 5 x 5 square. To highlight the ages and periods when Italian male and female mortality were roughly equal, Figure 25(b) presents a modified version of this map in which only three contour lines are drawn, for equal male and female probabilities of death and for levels 10% above and below equality. The two figures reveal the worsening discrepancy between male and female mortality. In 1887, male and female probabilities of death were roughly comparable at most ages, female mortality tending to be somewhat higher than male mortality before age 45 and male mortality tending to be somewhat higher than female mortality at older ages. By 1986, female mortality was substantially less than male mortality at all ages, being only half as high as male mortality between ages 15 and 70.

Two further ratio surfaces are presented in Figures 26 and 27. Figure 26 displays the ratio of Italian male mortality to French male mortality from age 10 to 70 for years 1900 to 1960. The ratio fluctuates busily, producing the large number of contour lines shown in Figure 26(a); in Figure 26(b) the surface is smoothed over weighted 5 x 5 squares. The two red rectangles reveal the greater toll of death among young French males relative to young Italian males during the two World Wars. The purple and blue shades on the bottom of the maps, under age 20 or so before World War I and after World War II, and under about age 35 between the wars, show when French males were experiencing less mortality than their Italian counterparts; at older ages, it is the Italians who had the advantage.

Figure 27 shows the difference, in the USA, between first and second birth rates, i.e., the proportion of all women of some age at some time who are having their first child minus the proportion who are having their second child. The most striking feature of the figure is the rapidity of the shift from the predominance of first births to the predominance of second births, as indicated by the dark horizontal swath giving way to a light swath. The midpoint of this shift is described by the contour at level zero running across the map at roughly age 25. The contour reaches a peak at age 30 in 1940 and falls to age 22 in 1960. In 1960, at the center of the baby boom, the shift from first births to second births is not only early, but also especially dramatic.

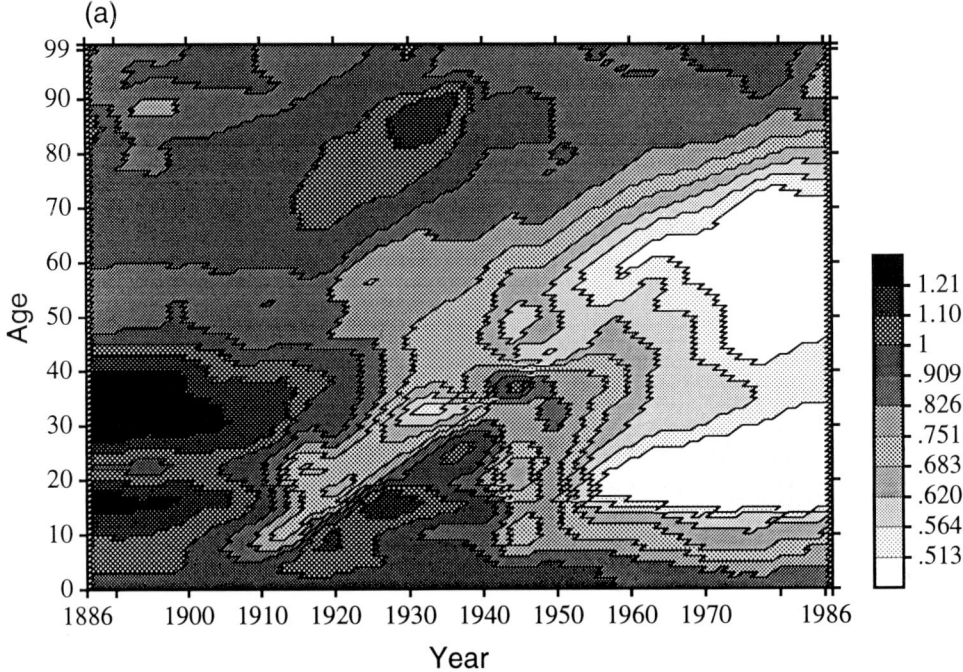

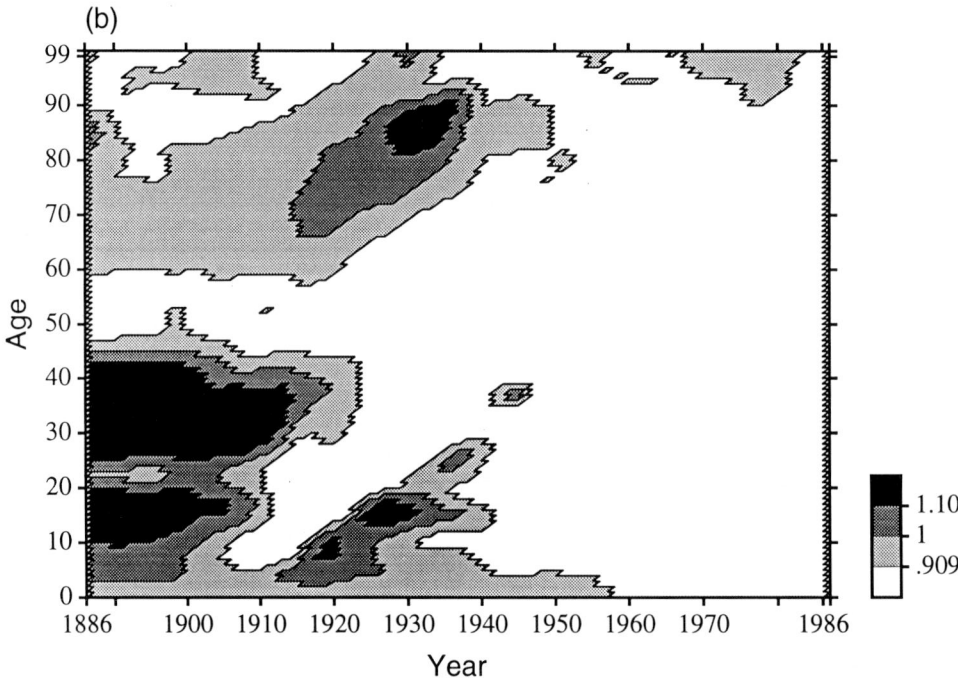

**Figure 25.** Italian female probabilities of death divided by Italian male probabilities of death, smoothed on a 5 x 5 square, and from age 0 to 99 and year 1886 to 1986: (a) with contour lines at multiples of 1.1 from 0.513 to 1.21; (b) with contour lines from 0.909 to 1.1.

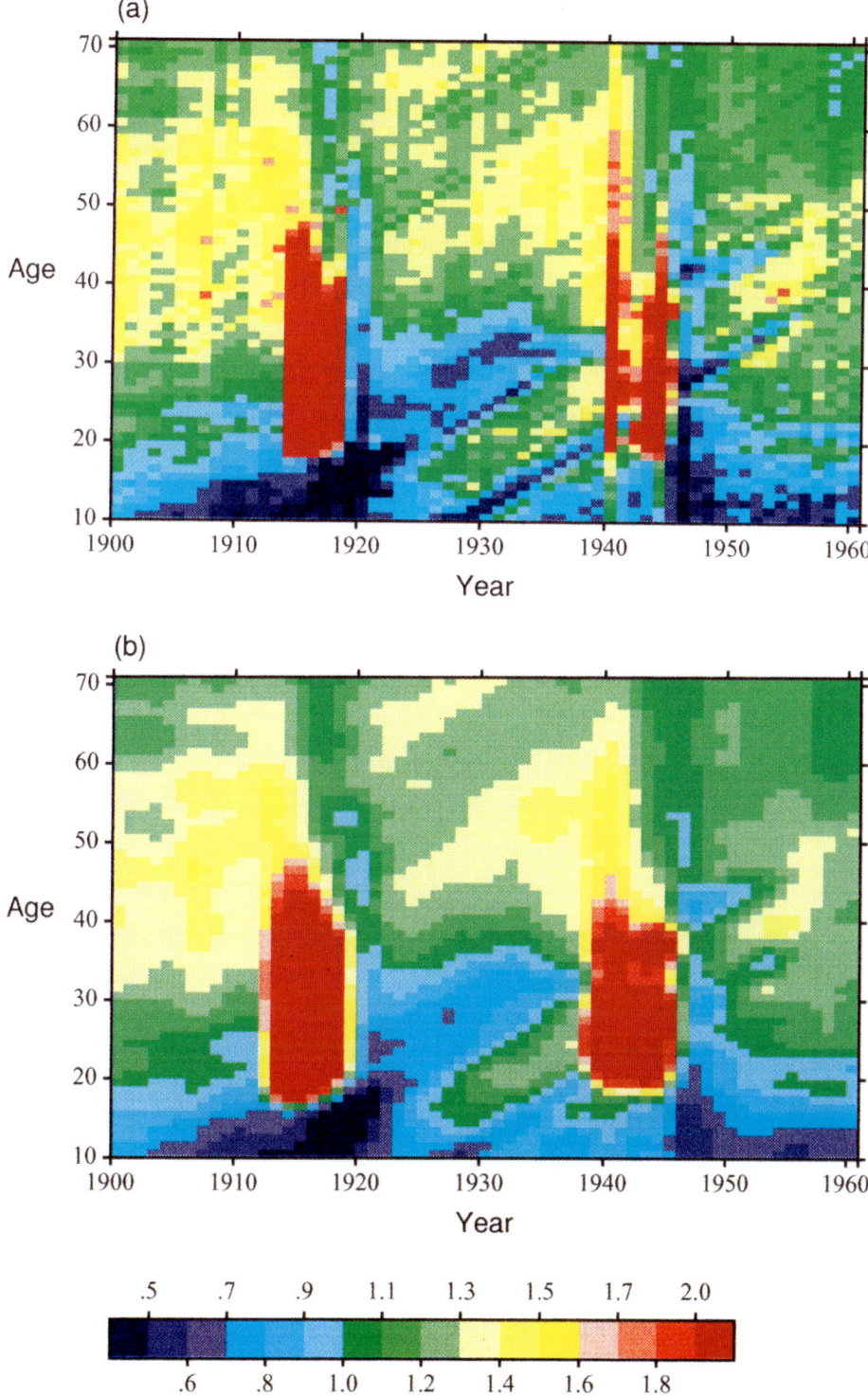

**Figure 26.** French male probabilities of death divided by Italian male probabilities of death (in color): (a) with contours selectively placed from 0.5 to 2.0 and from age 10 to 70 and year 1900 to 1960; and (b) as Figure 26(a), but smoothed on a weighted 5 x 5 square.

# 13. Sex-ratios, nuptiality, and cause-specific mortality

In addition to maps of death rates, birth rates and population levels, contour maps can be drawn based on any other kind of data that is structured along two dimensions. Figures 28, 29, and 30 suggest three possibilities. Figure 28 displays the ratio of females to males in Belgium, based on Veys'(1983) data. An interesting contour to follow on the map is the contour at level 1: at ages below this line, males outnumber females, and at older ages females predominate. The line starts at age 32 in 1892, rapidly falls to age 20 during World War I, gradually rises to age 43 or so by the mid-1940s, and then remains at roughly this age up through 1977. A striking feature of the map as a whole is the increasing predominance of females at older ages. Even in 1892, there were 25% more females than males at age 85, but by 1977, there were close to twice as many females at this age than males.

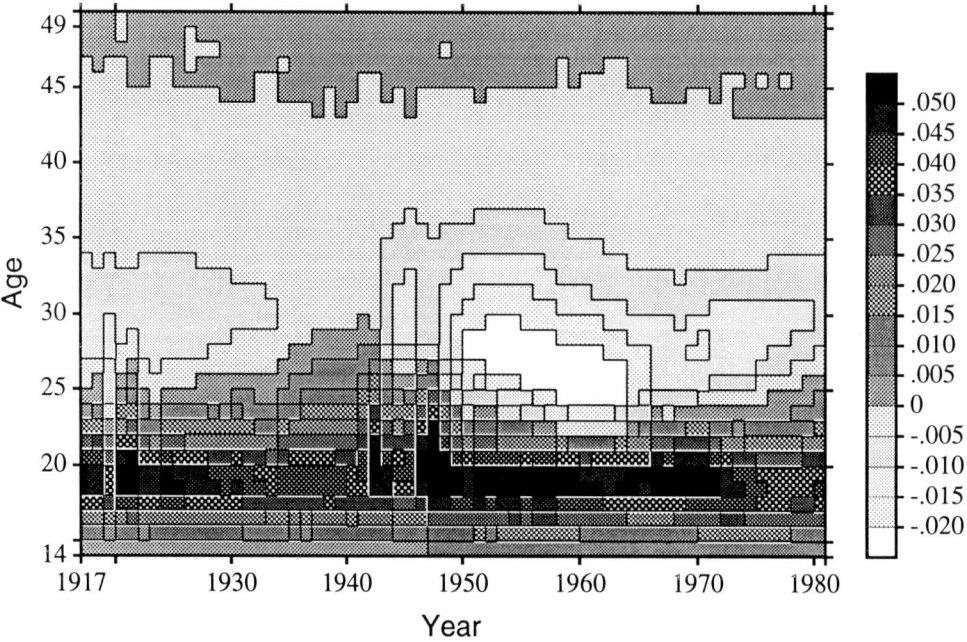

**Figure 27.** US birth rates at parity 1 minus those at parity 2, with contour lines from -0.02 to 0.05 at intervals of 0.005, and from age 14 to 49 and year 1917 to 1980.

Figure 29 shows age-specific marriage rates for Chinese females, based on Zeng et al. (1985, 1994). The rates in Figure 29(a) give the proportion of women at different ages and times who marry; the denominator is not the number of unmarried women but the total number of women. The rates in Figure 29(b), on the other hand, are conditional first marriage rates: the denominator is the number of unmarried women. Since the conditional rates were somewhat noisy, we smoothed them on a weighted 3 x 3 square.

The most striking pattern on the Lexis map in Figure 29(a) is the shift upward in age of first marriage. It is apparent from the map that marriage in China is concentrated in a short period of age. Consider, for example, the ages when female first marriage rates exceed 7.5%, i.e., the ages colored in yellow and red. The period of high marriage rates shifted from ages 15 through 20 in the early 1950s, to ages 18 through 21 in 1970, to ages 20 through 25 in 1980 and to ages 19 through 24 in 1987. As a result of this shift, the proportion of women who marry at age 17 fell from close to 20% in 1950 to about 2% around 1980, whereas the proportion who marry at age 23 rose from 2% to about 20%.

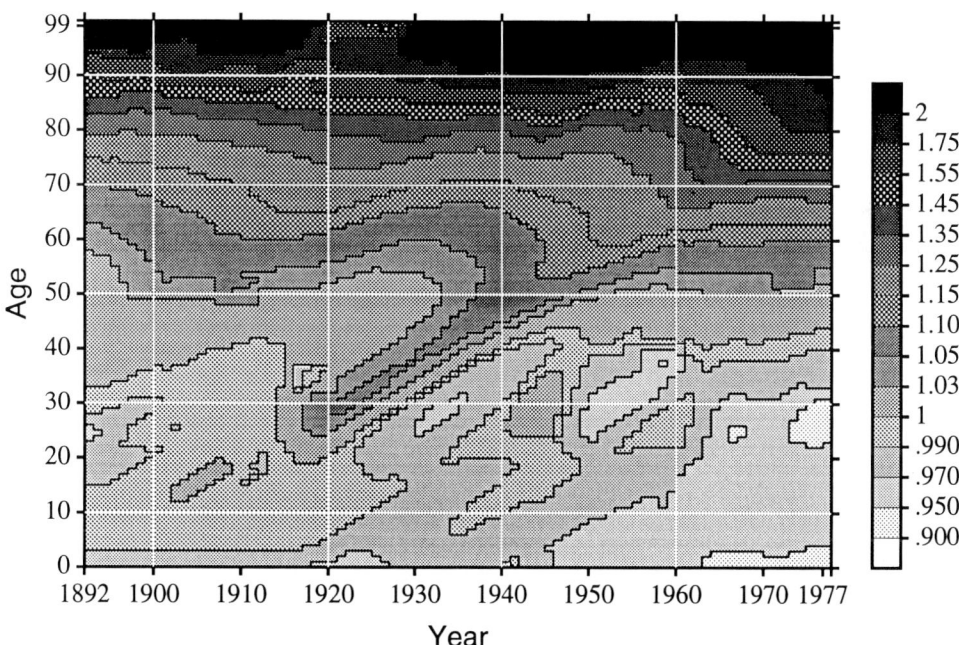

**Figure 28.** Belgian female population divided by Belgian male population, with contour lines selectively placed from 0.90 to 2.00, smoothed on a 5 x 5 square, with a grid, and from age 0 to 99 and year 1892 to 1977.

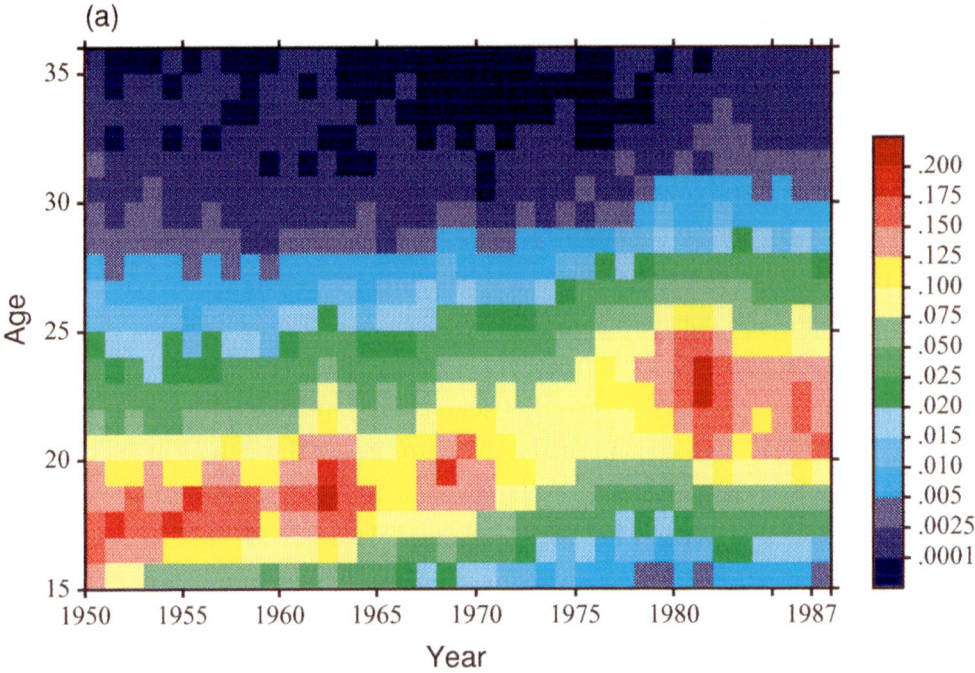

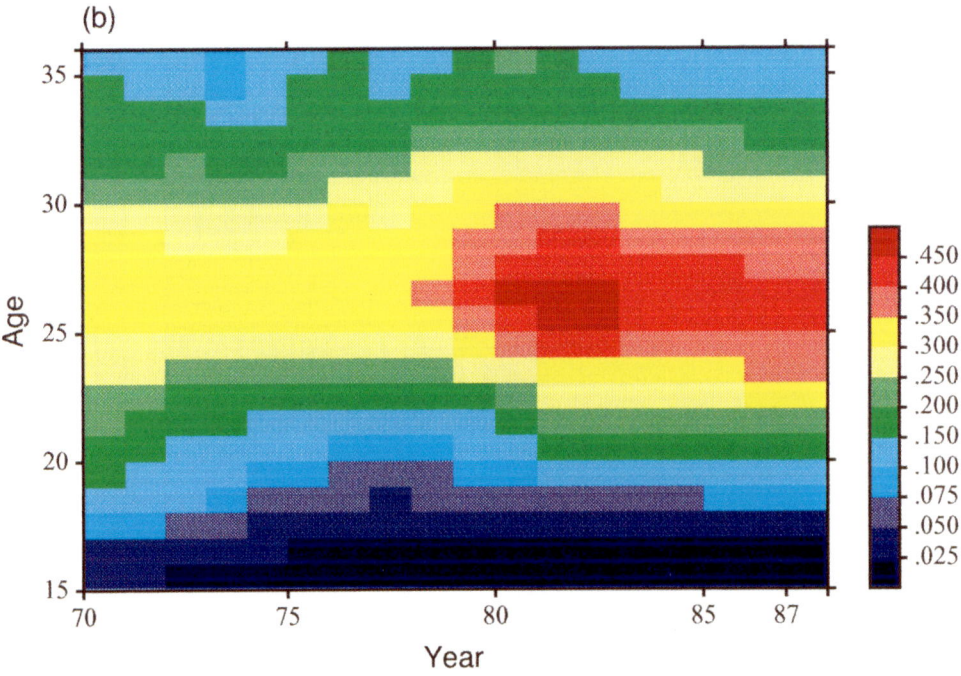

**Figure 29.** Chinese female first marriage rates (in color): (a) with contours selectively placed from 0.0001 to 0.2 and from age 15 to 35 and year 1950 to 1987; (b) smoothed and conditional (see text), with contours selectively placed from 0.025 to 0.45, from age 15 to 35 and year 1970 to 1987.

The yellow and red areas on the map in Figure 29(b) represent ages and years when more than a quarter of the unmarried women married. The tremendous spurt in marriages after 1979 of women in their mid and late 20s who had delayed marriage is marked by a dramatic red splotch. Among the cohort of women born in 1955, more than 40% of those who were still unmarried in 1980 (at age 25) married and more than 45% of the remainder married in 1981: more than two-thirds of the women who were not married at the start of the two-year period were married by the end of it.

Comparison of Figures 29(a) and 29(b) reveals some interesting differences between the patterns of unconditional and conditional marriage rates. Since the conditional rates equal the unconditional rates divided by the proportion never married, the conditional rates have to be higher than the unconditional rates. Nonetheless, it is somewhat startling how much higher they are, especially at older ages. The durable pattern of universal marriage in China implies that women in their late 20s who are not married as yet have a high chance of marrying. Consider age 25 through 30, for instance. A swatch of yellow and red shades runs across Figure 29(b), indicating conditional

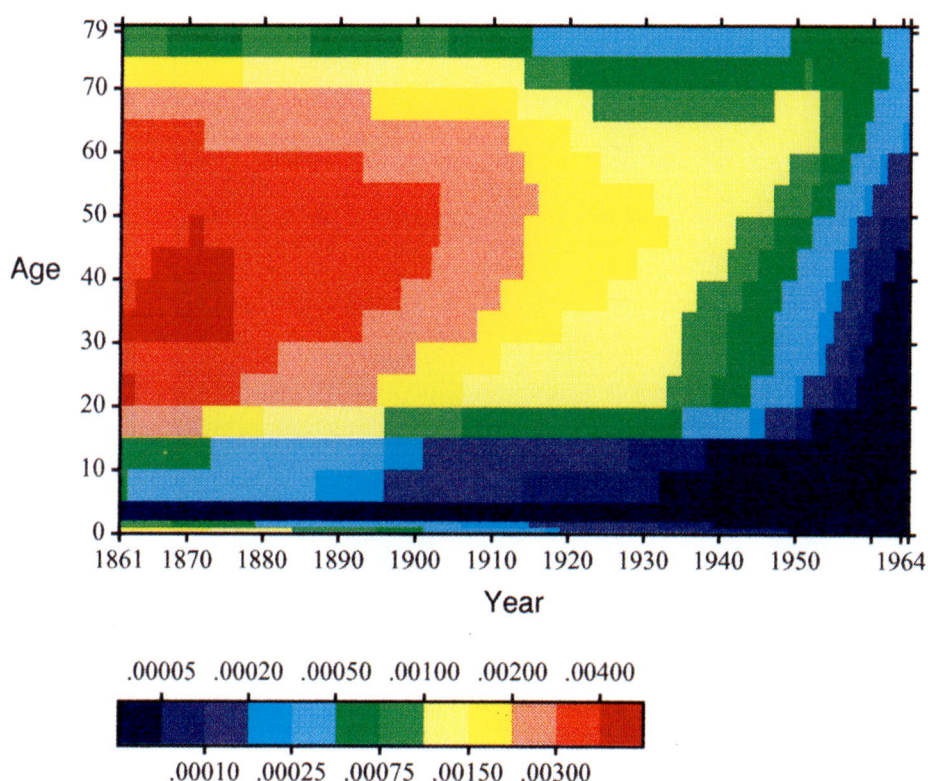

**Figure 30.** Death rates from tuberculosis for English and Welsh males (in color), with contours from 0.00005 to 0.004, and from age 0 to 79 and year 1861 to 1964.

marriage rates above 25% For every cohort shown on the map, at least 80% of the women who were not married at age 25 were married by age 30.

Contour maps can also be used to display surfaces of cause-specific mortality. In Figure 30, for instance, male mortality in England and Wales from tuberculosis is displayed for 80 years of age over about a century of time; the map is based on interpolations of data from Keyfitz and Flieger (1968). The high toll of mortality exacted by tuberculosis in the middle of ages of life, especially from 30 to 60, is apparent on the map, as is the acceleration of progress against tuberculosis after World War II. This progress was very rapid, with probabilities of death at age 40, for instance, falling from 1 in 1,000 in 1940 to 1 in 20,000 in 1963. Note also that there seems to be some evidence of cohort effects interacting with the period trend.

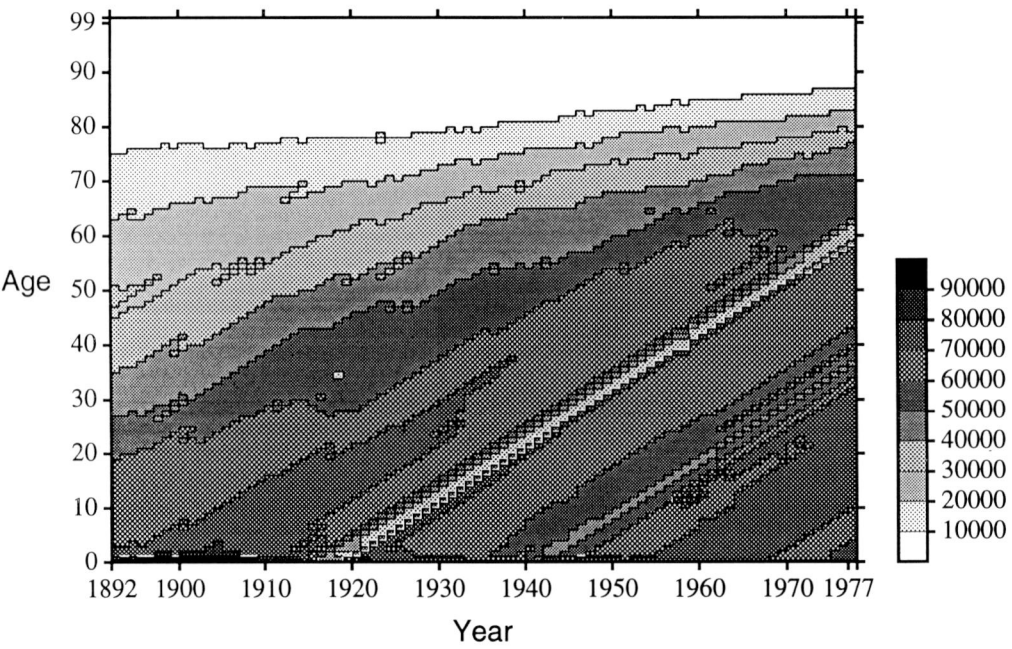

**Figure 31.** Belgian female population for single year of age and time, with contour lines from 10000 to 90000 at intervals of 10000, and from age 0 to 99 and year 1892 to 1977.

# 14. Life table statistics for Belgian females

Life tables often provide statistics by age and over time on population size, number of deaths, death rates, period survivorship, period life expectancy, and sometimes cohort survivorship. All six of these statistics are available, for example, in Veys' (1983) compilation of Belgian life tables from age 0 to 99 for years 1892 to 1977. Figures 31 through 36 use Vey's data for Belgian females to illustrate the different kinds of contour map patterns produced by different kinds of life table statistics. The differences in the patterns are quite striking, each kind of population statistic producing what might be called its characteristic pattern, fingerprint, or signature:

(1)  Lexis surfaces of population levels (Figure 31) tend to show strong diagonals at younger ages, bending over toward horizontal lines at advanced ages.

(2)  Surfaces of deaths (Figure 32) tend to be marked by two ridges running over time, one ridge (a cliff, really) highest in infancy, the other highest around age 70 or 80. As progress is made against mortality, the first ridge declines, but the second rises: deaths become increasingly concentrated around age 80. Perpendicular ridges mark periods of devastation, most notably World War I and its aftermath for Belgium.

(3)  Surfaces of mortality (Figure 33) are characterized by a valley between two steep walls of high mortality in infancy and at advanced ages. Again, perpendicular ridges mark disasters. Over time, as progress is made against mortality, the valley slopes off, most rapidly at younger ages, producing contours that sometimes look like a flattened S and sometimes like a U turned sideways.

(4)  Survivorship (Figures 34 and 36) and life expectancy (Figure 35) fall off with age, more slowly in recent years because of the progress that has been made against mortality.

The maps of survivorship and life expectancy tend to be smoother than the maps of deaths and mortality rates, the life expectancy maps being the smoothest. This is to be expected: life expectancy can be considered a kind of average of survivorship figures, and survivorship an average of death rates. Moreover, the cohort maps tend to be smoother than the period maps, since the cohort maps average out period effects.

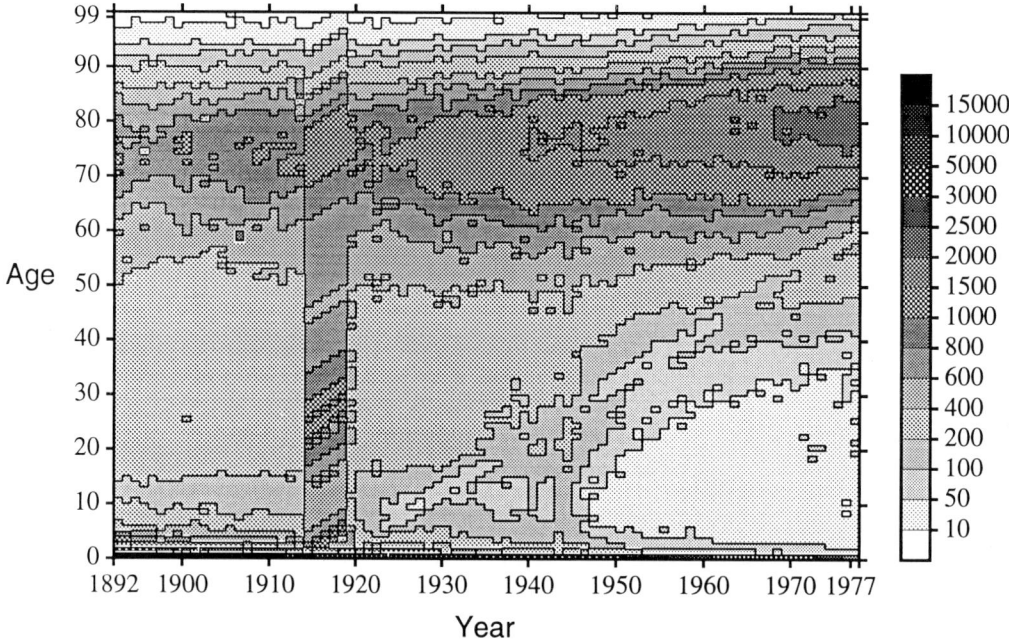

**Figure 32.** Belgian female deaths, with contour lines selectively placed from 10 to 15,000, and from age 0 to 99 and year 1892 to 1977.

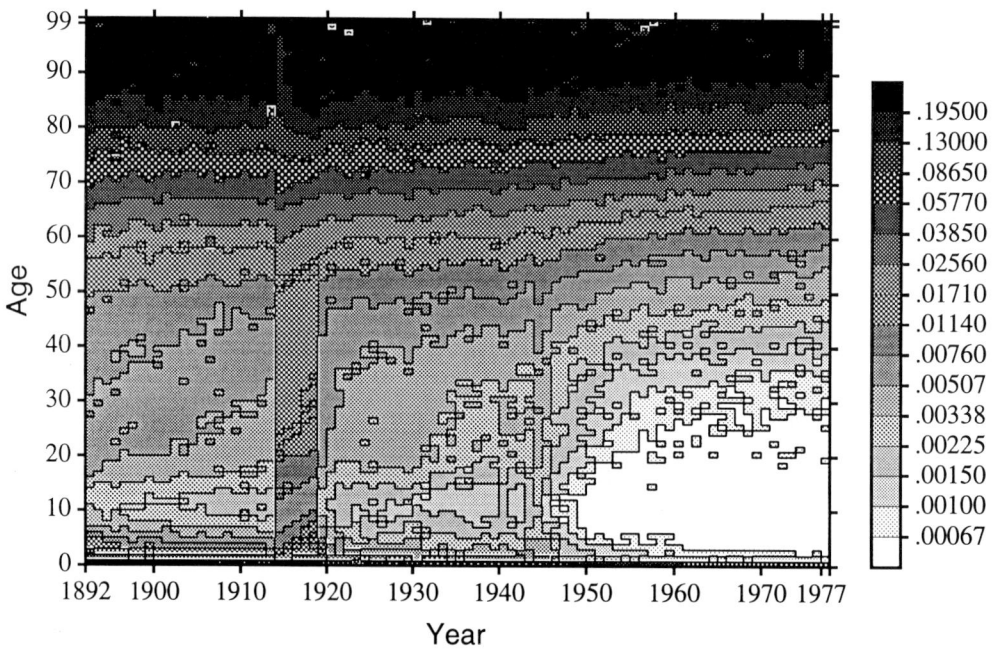

**Figure 33.** Probabilities of death for Belgian females, with contour lines from 0.000667 to 0.195 at multiples of 1.5, and from age 0 to 99 and year 1892 to 1977.

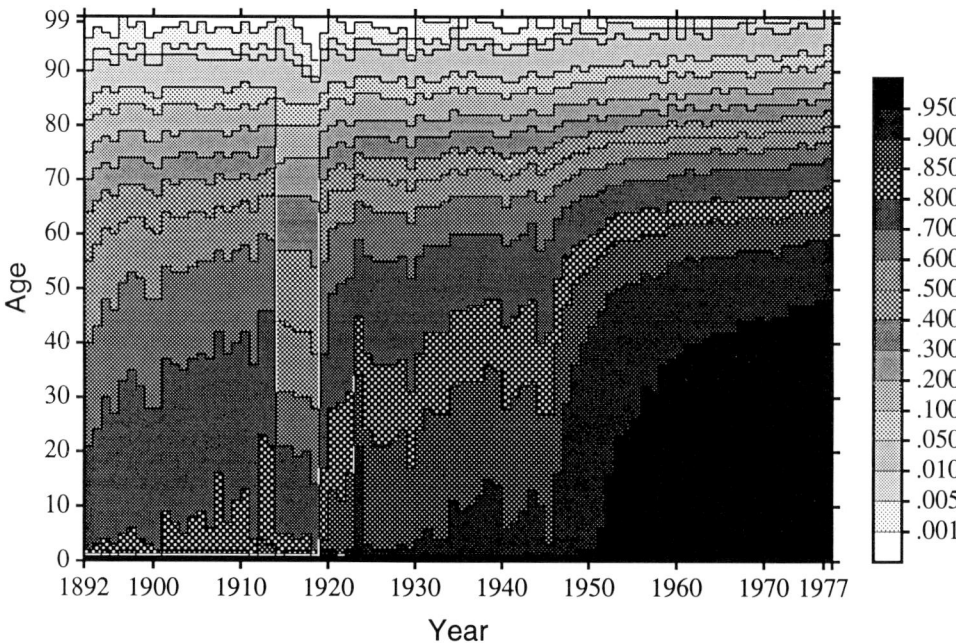

**Figure 34.** Belgian female period survivorship, with contour lines selectively placed from 0.001 to 0.95, from age 0 to 99 and year 1892 to 1977.

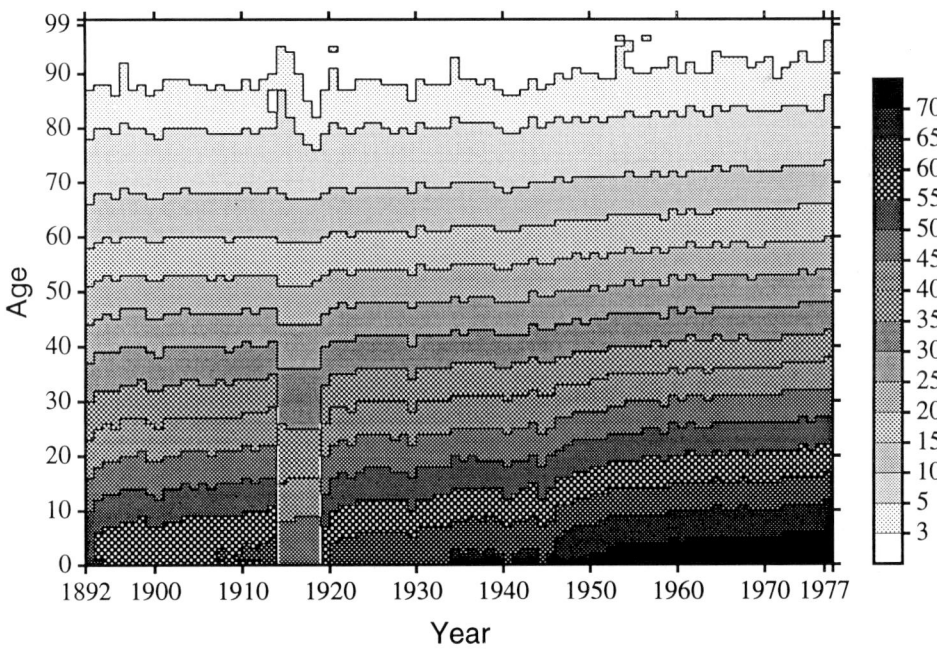

**Figure 35.** Belgian female period life expectancy, with contour lines selectively placed from 3 to 70, from age 0 to 99 and year 1892 to 1977.

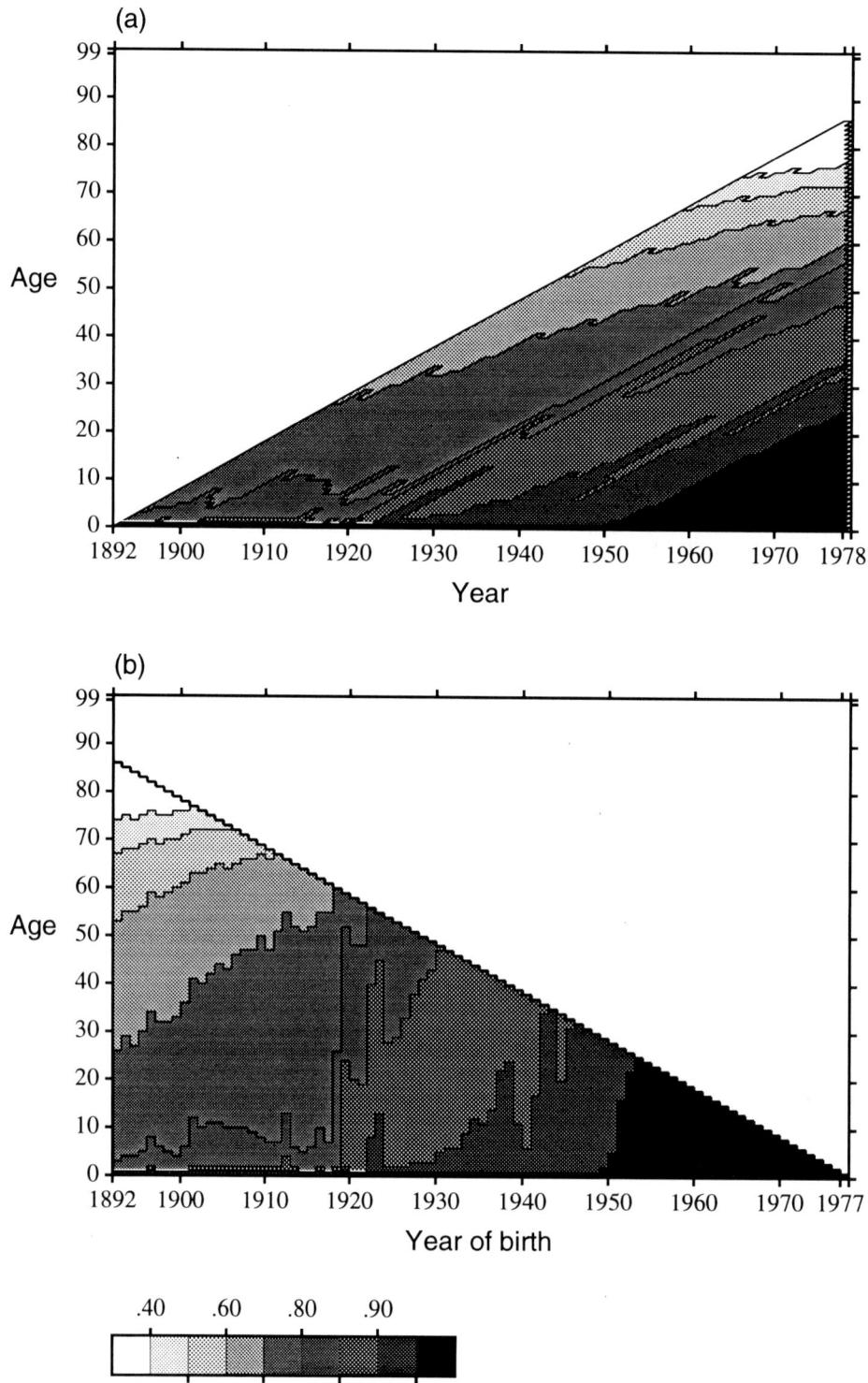

**Figure 36.** Belgian female cohort survivorship, with contour lines selectively placed from 0.4 to 0.95, from age 0 to 99 and year 1892 to 1977: (a) by current year and age; (b) by year of birth and age.

# 15. U.S. female mortality 1900-2050

Faber (1982) published life tables for US males and females by single year of age from birth to 119 for every tenth year from 1900 through 2050. The mortality estimates at advanced ages and after 1980 are based on extrapolations. Figure 37 displays the surface of the force of mortality for US males and females up through age 84. Note that the Lexis map graphically reveals Faber's underlying assumption that progress against mortality will slow down in the future.

Some implications of the assumptions underlying Faber's projections are presented in Figure 38, which displays the force of mortality over age relative to the force of mortality in 1980. The right side of Figure 38 does not mirror the left side. The left side shows the rapid historical progress that has been achieved in reducing mortality at most ages and the acceleration of progress at some ages, especially some of the older ages. The right side portrays a lacklustre future, with slow and slowing rates of progress. Perhaps Faber's forecasts can be described as "conservative" in some sense, but they are certainly radically different from the performance of the past.

# 16. Oldest-old mortality

As shown earlier in Figures 12 and 13, the numbers of octogenarians, nonagenarians, and centenarians has exploded in recent decades. Close to half of female deaths and a third of male deaths in developed countries now occur among those above age 80. To help meet the need for more extensive, more reliable data on mortality and survival at advanced ages, the Odense Archive of Population Data on Aging was established in 1992 at Odense University Medical School.

An important part of the archive is the Kannisto-Thatcher Oldest-Old Database. Väinö Kannisto, Distinguished Research Fellow at Odense University Medical School and former United Nations advisor on demographic and social statistics, assembled the core set of data, tested the data for quality, and converted the data into cohort mortality histories. These data, which pertain to death counts and population counts by year of age, year of birth, and current year over the last four decades or so in some thirty countries, permit estimation of death rates after age 80. Also included in the database are comparable materials on England and Wales made available by A. Thatcher, former

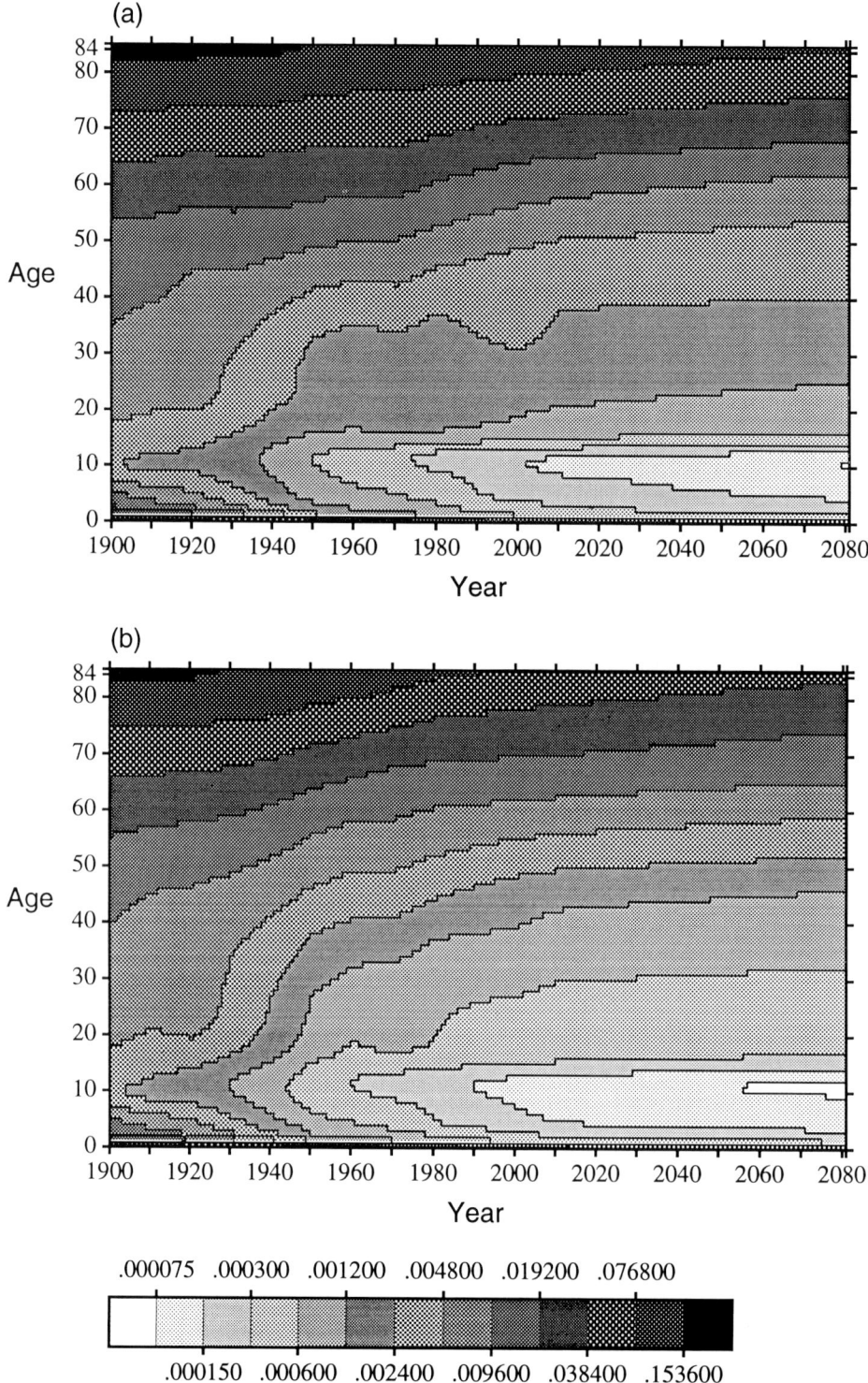

**Figure 37.** Force of mortality for US (a) males and (b) females based on Faber (1982) life tables, with contour lines from 0.000075 to 0.1536 at multiples of 2, and from age 0 to 84 and year 1900 to 2080.

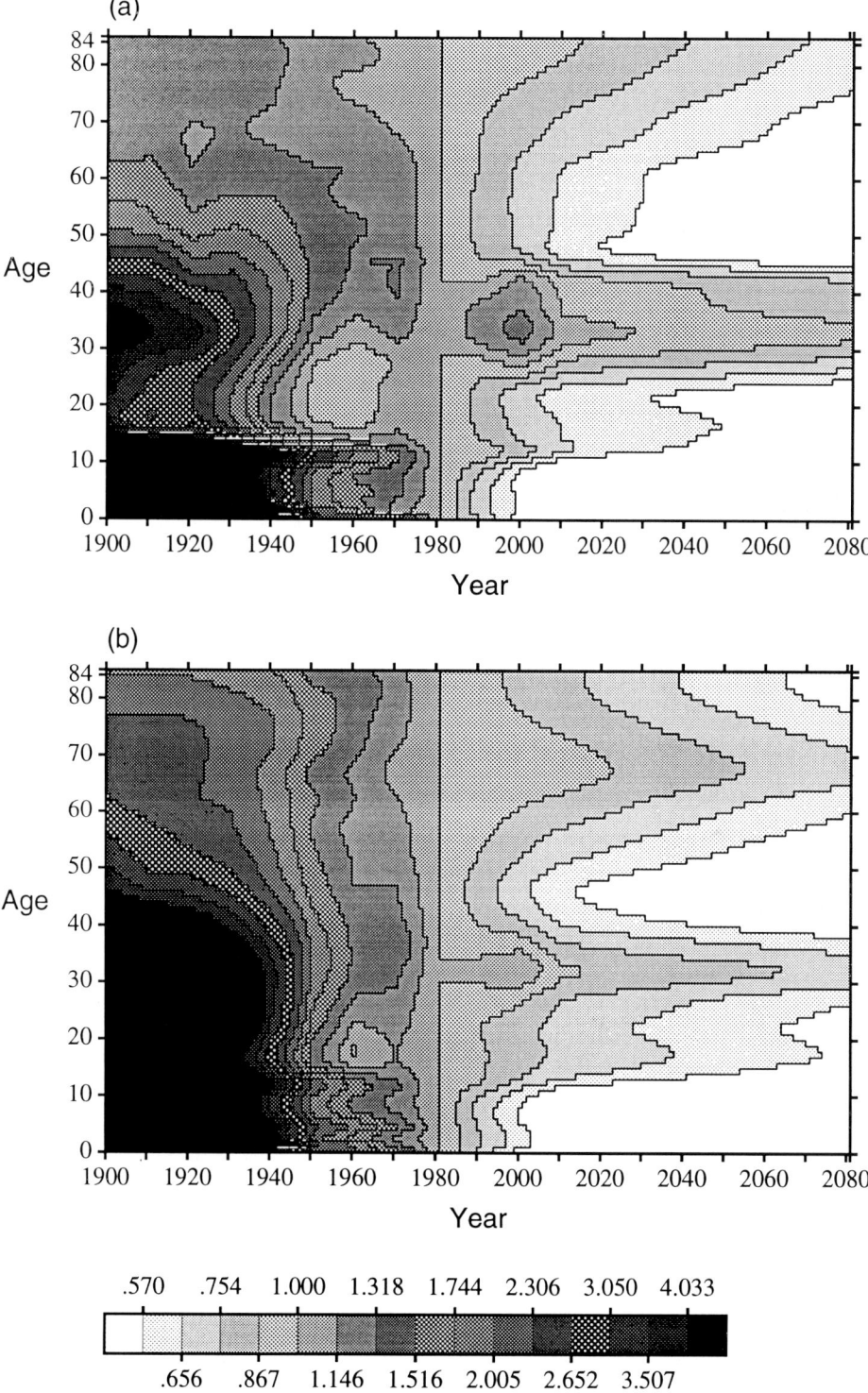

**Figure 38.** Force of mortality for US (a) males and (b) females relative to 1980 age-specified levels, with contour lines from 0.570 to 4.033 at multiples of 1.146, and from age 0 to 84 and year 1900 to 2080.

Director of the Office of Population Censuses and Surveys and Registrar-General of England and Wales. Kannisto and Thatcher used the same extinct-cohort method to estimate population counts from death counts.

In addition, the Odense Archive includes an exceptionally reliable database of death counts and population counts for Sweden, from 1861 until the present, starting at age 50. This database was created by Hans Lundström, a demographer at Statistics Sweden. Data from the Odense Archive have been analyzed in four other monographs in this series and will undoubtedly be used in future monographs as well. The four monographs are by Kannisto (1996), Jeune and Vaupel (1995), Kannisto (1995), and Thatcher et al. (forthcoming). The next figures in this monograph, Figures 39 through 44, are based on data from the Odense Archive--from Lundström's database for Sweden and from the Kannisto-Thatcher Oldest-Old database for other countries.

Figure 39 displays the evolution of mortality after age 80 since 1861 for females and males in Sweden. Because the underlying data are broken down by both year of birth and current year, the surfaces consists of small triangles. The mortality levels are estimates of the force of mortality: they are very nearly equal to death rates calculated by dividing the number of deaths in a triangle by the person-years lived in the triangle.

The grey diagonals at the top of the figures represent the lingering survival of the last member of a cohort: the red triangle at the end of the diagonal marks the death of the exceptional longliver. Since 1861 longevity records have been repeatedly broken. In the 1860s and 1870s an occasional female survived to 105 and an occasional male to 101. In the 1980s a woman died at age 111 and in 1991 a man was still alive at 108. The contour lines tend to move upward to more advanced ages over time: this reflects improvements in mortality. For 80-year-old females in the 1860s, the force of mortality was about 0.15. In the 1980s it had fallen to under 0.06 and it was not until age 89 that the force of mortality reached 0.15. Most of this progress was achieved since the 1930s. For males the improvements in mortality are less dramatic but still apparent.

Figures 40, 41 and 42 presents similar data on the same mortality-rate scale but in black and white. The data for England and Wales in Fig. 40 start in 1911. The data for Japan in Fig. 41 start in 1950. Finally, data for an aggregate of 13 countries from 1950 through 1990 are presented in Fig. 42. The 13 countries are Austria, Denmark, England and Wales, Finland, France, Germany (West), Iceland, Italy, Japan, the Netherlands, Norway, Sweden, and Switzerland. As explained in Kannisto (1994), these countries have particularly reliable data that is available for all or most of the period 1950-1990.

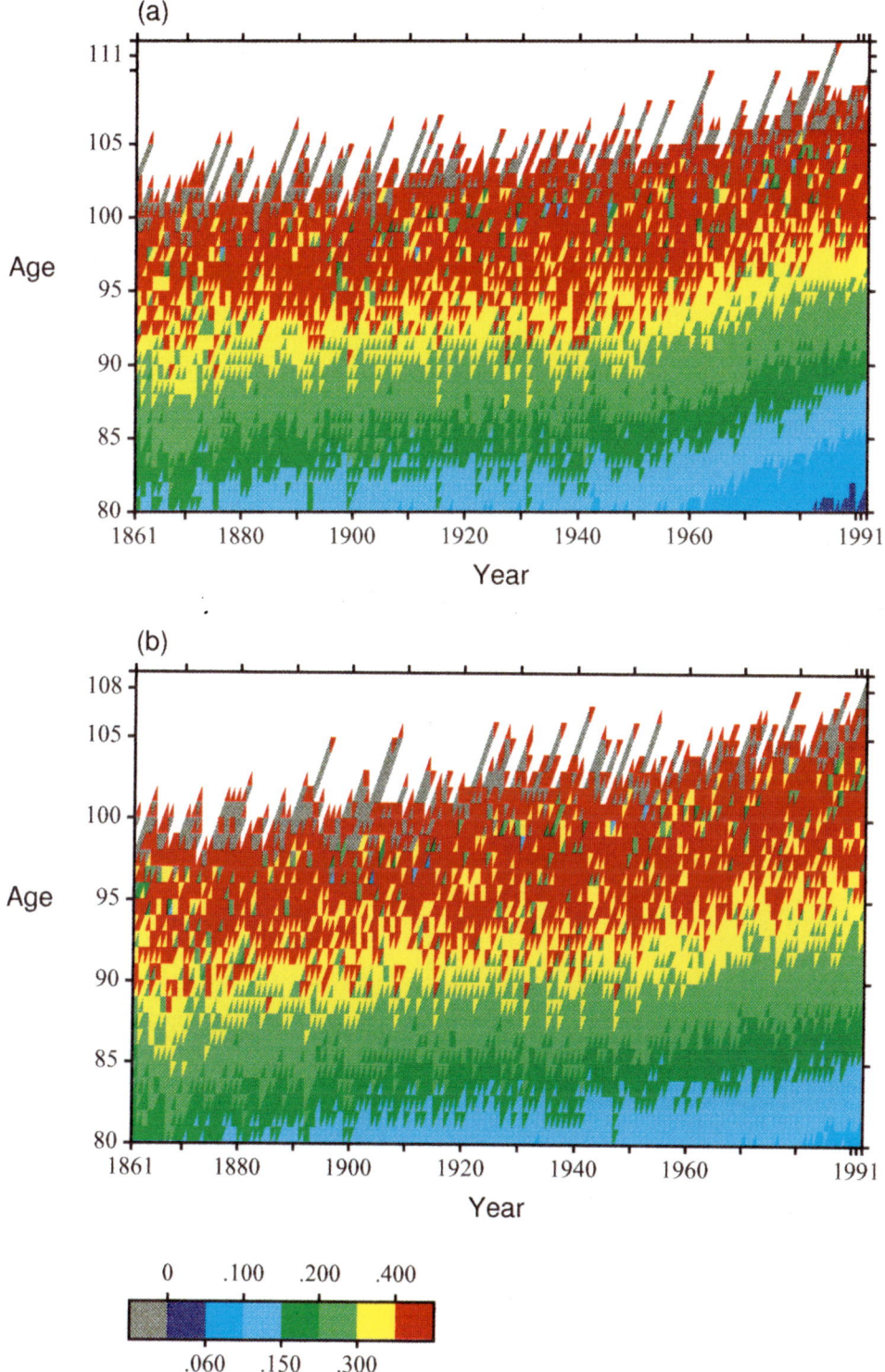

**Figure 39.** Force of mortality in Sweden (in color), with contours placed from 0 to 0.4: (a) female, from age 80 to 111 and year 1861 to 1991; (b) male, from age 80 to 108 and year 1861 to 1991.

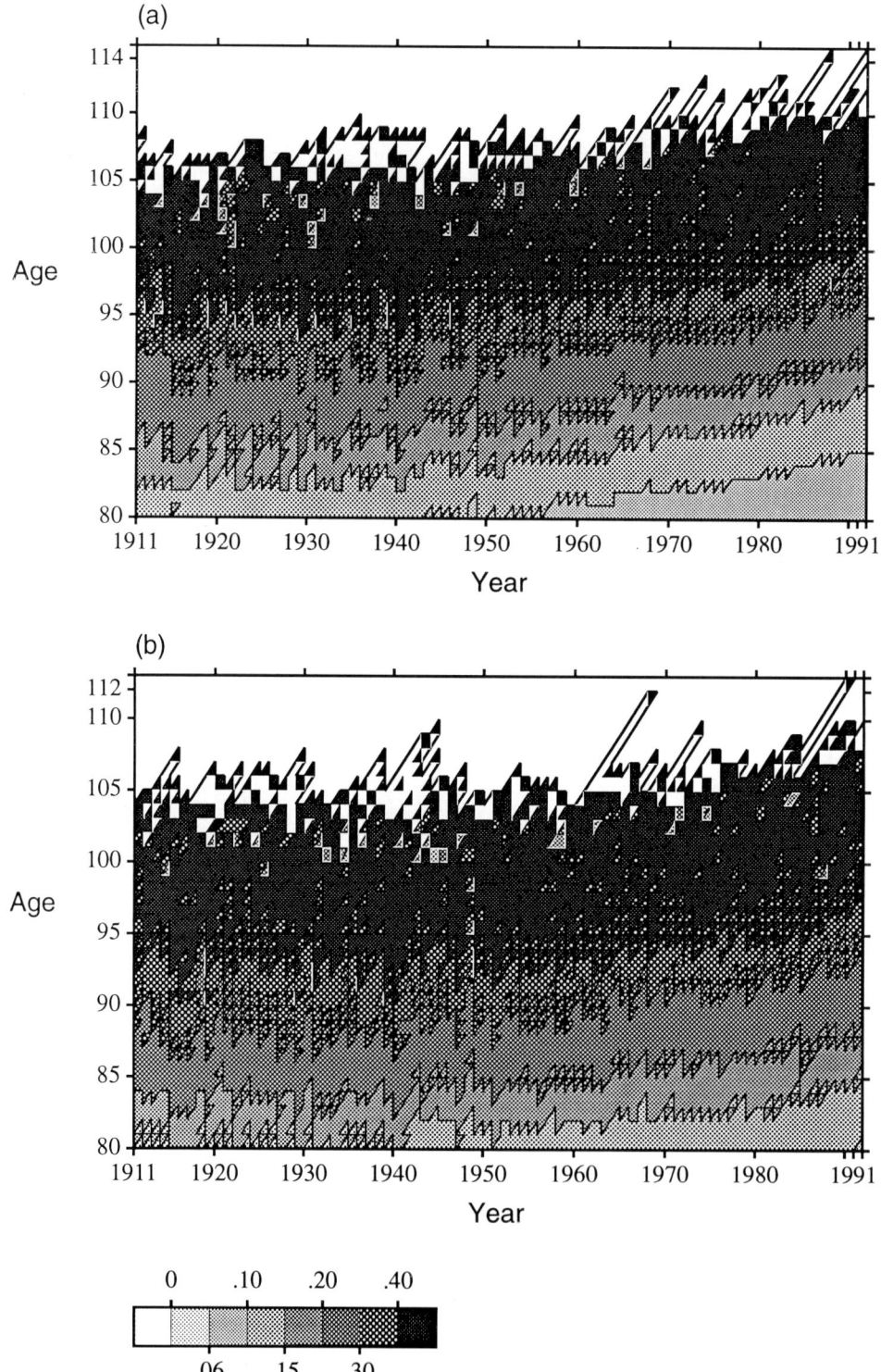

**Figure 40.** Force of mortality in England and Wales, with contour lines placed from 0 to 0.4: (a) female, from age 80 to 114 and year 1911 to 1991; (b) male, from age 80 to 112 and year 1911 to 1991.

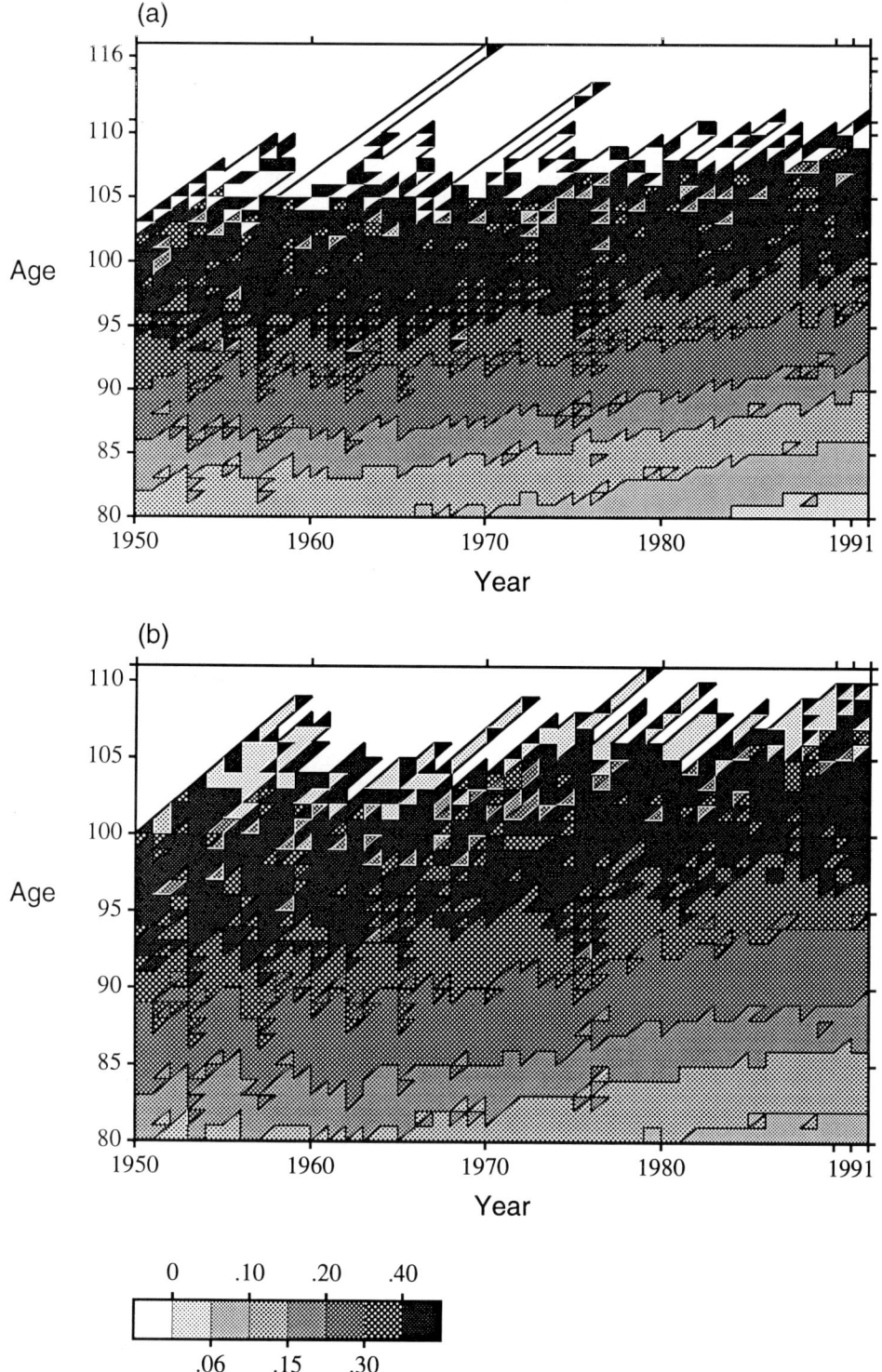

**Figure 41.** Force of mortality in Japan, with contour lines placed from 0 to 0.4: (a) female, from age 80 to 116 and year 1950 to 1991; (b) male, from age 80 to 110 and year 1950 to 1991.

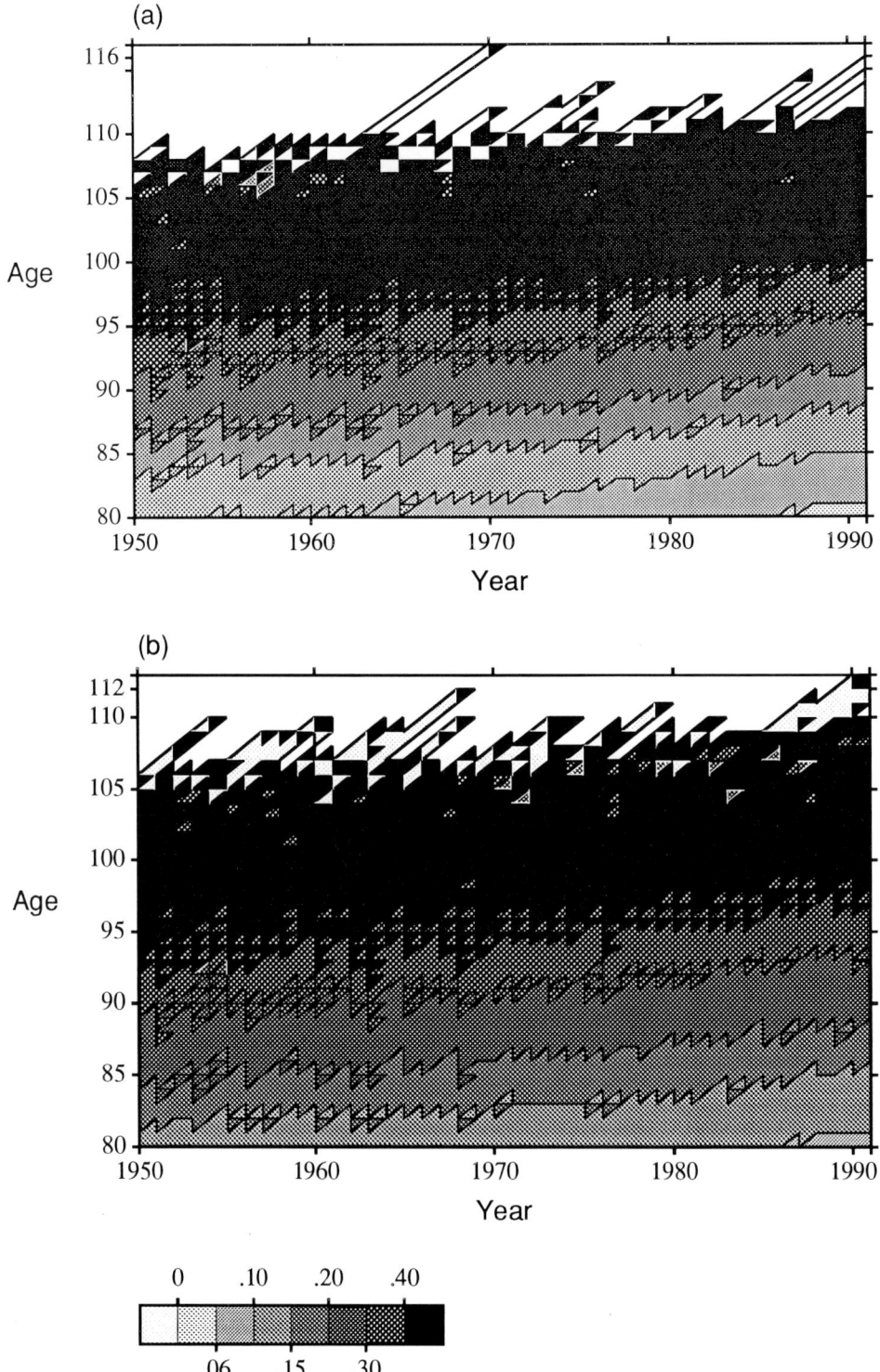

**Figure 42.** Force of mortality in aggregate of 13 countries, with contour lines selectively placed from 0 to 0.4: (a) female, from age 80 to 116 and year 1950 to 1990; (b) male, from age 80 to 112 and year 1950 to 1990.

For females the death rate reaches 0.15 at age 82 or 83 at the start of all three maps and reaches age 89 or 90 in 1990 or 1991. Indeed, comparison of the various mortality levels shows that by 1990 Sweden, England and Wales, Japan, and the aggregate of 13 countries had roughly similar trajectories of mortality after age 80, both for females and for males. More detailed comparisons of similarities and differences are provided by Kannisto (1996).

As discussed in Jeune and Vaupel (1995), many reputed centenarians are actually much younger and genuine supercentenarians (age 110 and above) may only have emerged in recent decades. Kannisto, Thatcher, and Lundström endeavored to check questionable longlivers, especially supercentenarians, and to remove cases that seemed doubtful. The Swedish database created by Lundström is exceptionally reliable, but even it may contain an error here and there at some ages and years. Data for other countries certainly include some errors that may be relatively large at the most advanced ages when hardly anyone is alive. Kannisto and Thatcher usually erred on the side of caution and removed people who may actually have attained an advanced age; more rarely they may have inadvertently accepted a dubious case. In particular, the Japanese woman who died at age 116 in 1970, as shown on both Fig. 41a and 42a, seems questionable. The second longest-lived member of her birth cohort died at age 104 and in both previous and subsequent birth cohorts record longevity was several years less, not only for Japan but for the aggregate of 13 countries as well.

# 17. Checking data quality

As briefly discussed by Kannisto (1994), demographers have developed a number of tests of the plausibility of population counts and death counts at older ages. One concern is with age-heaping, the tendency in some countries and times for ages to be rounded off. Age for some 88-year-olds or for some 91-year-olds might, for instance, be given as 90. Another concern is with age-exaggeration. Lexis maps can provide some help to demographers in checking for systematic errors or deficiencies in large bodies of data that may pertain to several decades of time and age. Figures 43 and 44 illustrate this.

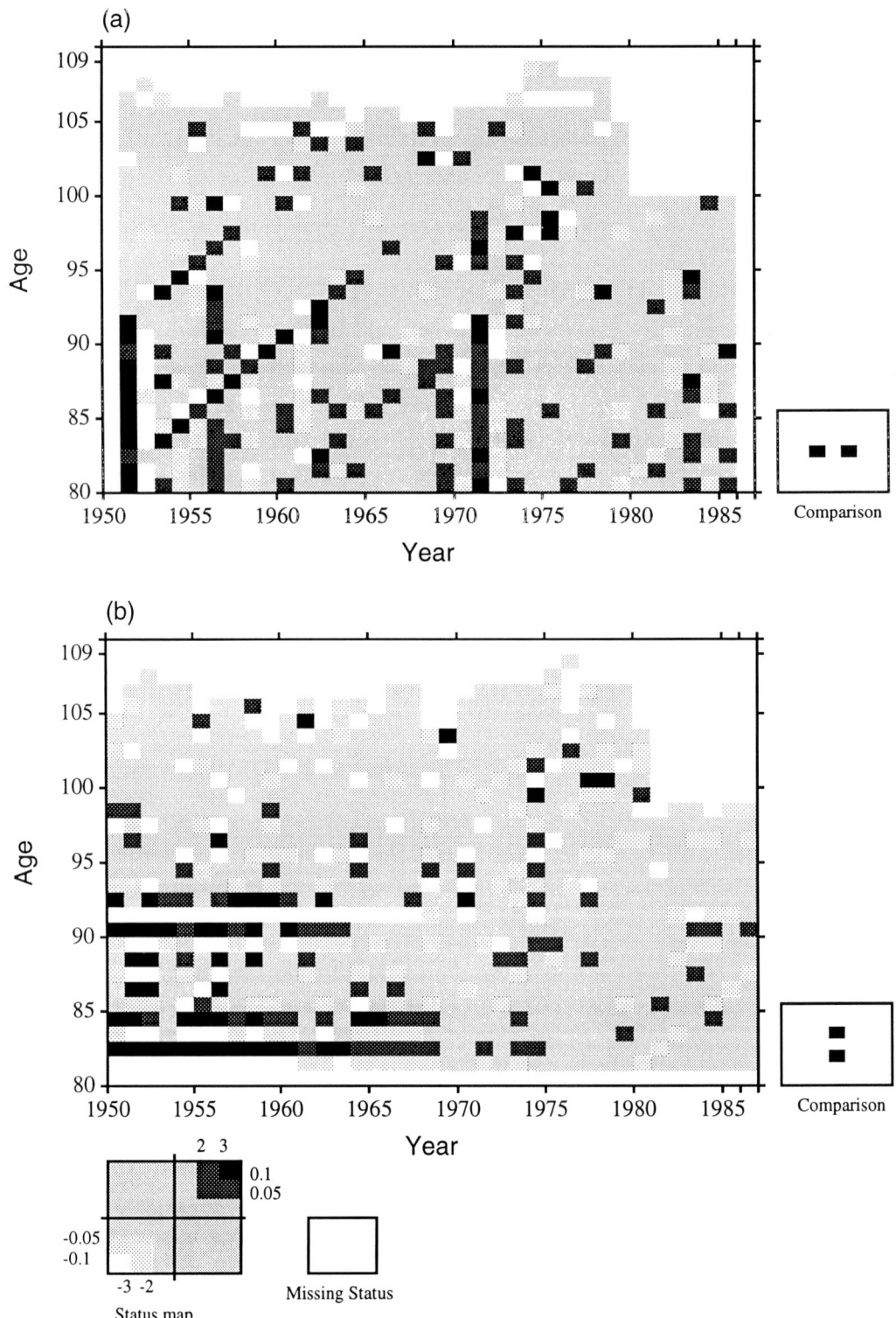

**Figure 43.** Data quality checks for Spanish males, from age 80 to 108 and year 1950 to 1986: (a) period comparison with adjacent years; (b) period comparison with adjacent ages.

The figures are based on an idea suggested by James Vaupel and developed by Kirill Andreev, a research statistician at Odense University's Aging Research Center. The basic idea is that death rates generally change slowly and smoothly over age and time. Hence, the death rate in a population at some age and in some year or cohort should usually be close to the average of the death rates at same age in adjacent years or cohorts and to the average of the death rates at adjacent ages in the same year or cohort.

As shown in Figure 1 and in other figures, an event such as World War I or the Spanish Influenza epidemic can produce a marked increase in mortality from one year to the next. Furthermore, as shown in Figures 39 to 42, at very high ages, when population sizes are small, random fluctuations can produce the appearance of rapid changes in death rates. To filter out such small-population noise, it might be stipulated that the death rate at some age and time will be considered suspect only if it is at least 2 or 3 standard deviations away from the average of the death rate for adjacent ages, times, or cohorts. However, population sizes may be so large at younger ages that such a rule might classify insubstantial mortality fluctuations as being suspect. Consequently, a second filter might also be used: the deviation of a death rate from the average of the neighboring rates might have to exceed, say, 5 or 10 percent of the average before the death rate is considered suspect.

Such rules were used to produce Figure 43, which pertains to data on death rates--as measured by the so-called central death rate, $m(x)$--for Spanish males above age 80 and between 1950 and 1986. In Figure 43a, the death rate at some age x and in some year is compared with the average of the death rates at ages x-1 and x+1 in the same year. As indicated in the small box labelled "status map", a very dark grey is used if a death rate is more than 3 standard deviations higher and more than 10 percent greater than the average of the adjacent rates. A somewhat less dark grey is used if a death is more than 2 standard deviations higher and more than 5 percent greater. Lighter shades of grey indicate death rates that are correspondingly too low.

The pattern in Figure 43b suggests that there were problems of age-heaping for Spanish males up through the late 1960s and perhaps even up to 1975 at ages below 100 and that there may have been problems at age 100 as well in the 1970s. (The white area in the top right corner of the map reflects the fact that data are not available after age 100 since 1981.) The database starts at age 80, so comparisons cannot be made at that age. At age 81, death rates appear too low compared with the average of the rates at 80 and 82. One possibility is that some deaths that actually occurred at age 81 were reported to occur at age 80. This would also help explain why death rates at age 82 appear to be too high. There may also be a tendency to favor reporting even rather than odd ages--82, 84, 86, 88, 90, and 92 stand out as ages with suspiciously high death rates.

88

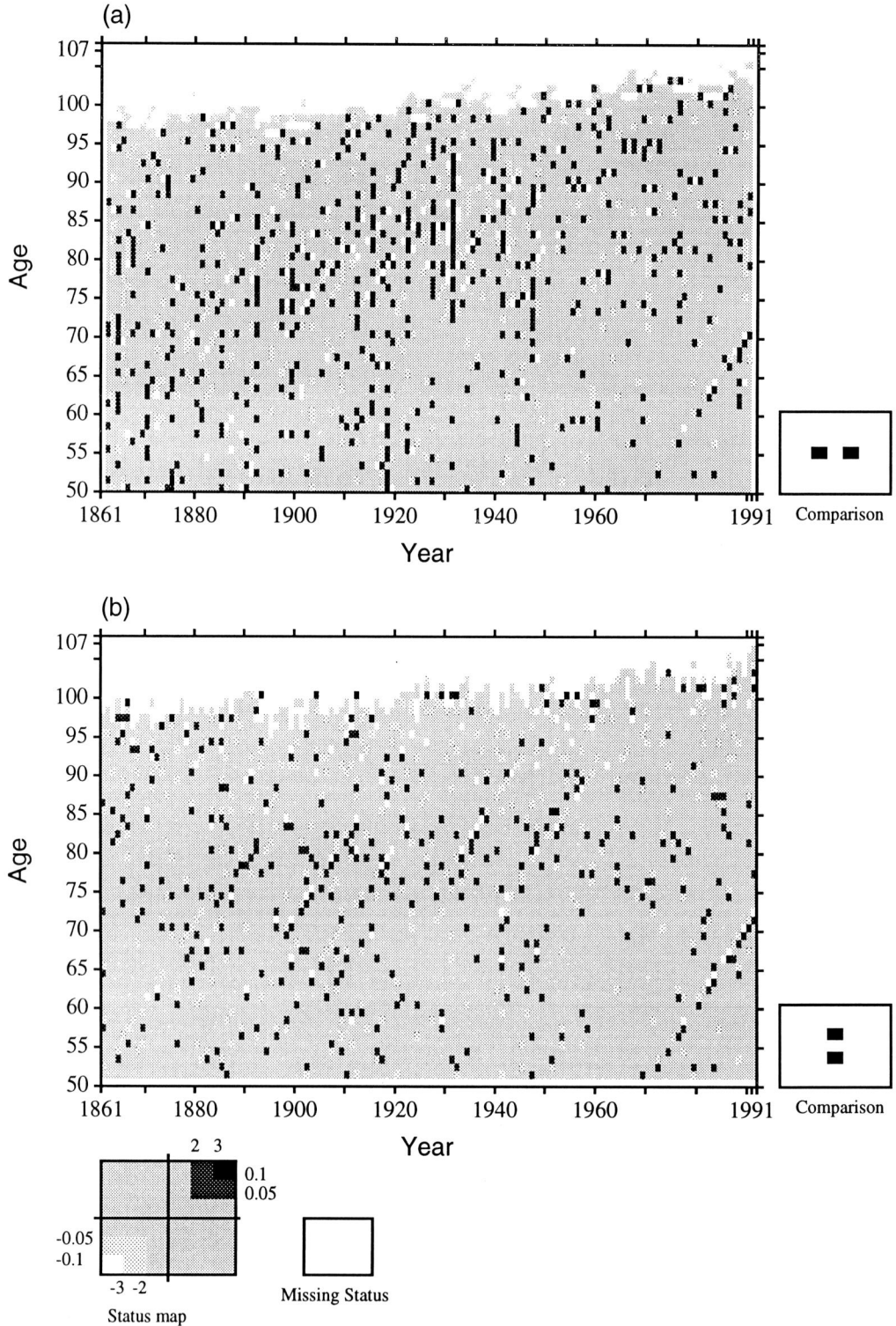

**Figure 44.** Data quality checks for Swedish males, from age 50 to 107 and year 1861 to 1991: (a) period comparison with adjacent years; (b) period comparison with adjacent ages.

In Figure 43a comparisons are made of death rates with the average of adjacent death rates at the same age but in the previous and following year. Some years, 1971 for instance, stand out as bad years. The map also reveals an intriguing cohort anomaly. The cohort that reached age 80 in 1950--that is, the cohort born in 1870--suffers excess mortality at most ages between 81 and 96. Similarly, the cohort that reached age 90 in 1950, the cohort born in 1860, suffers excess mortality at most ages 91 and 97. This could be explained by a tendency to round off year-of-birth on death certificates.

Figure 44 present comparable maps for Swedish males, but for a much longer time period--from 1861 through 1991--and starting at age 50 rather than 80. There is no evidence of age-heaping in Figure 44b. There are some period effects in Figure 44a, such as the elevation of mortality in 1918, especially among males in their 50s, due to the Spanish Influenza, as well as an intriguing elevation of death rates after age 70 in 1932. In both Figure 44a and 44b there are some diagonal, cohort patterns. The most striking of these diagonals suggests persistently low mortality for people born in 1919 compared with people born in 1920.

# 18. High Danish mortality

Danish life expectancy used to be among the highest in the world; now it falls below that in many other developed countries. Current Danish mortality, expecially for people in their 30s through 60s, tends to be relatively high compared with mortality in Sweden, Norway, the Netherlands, and various other countries. This unfavorable development has excited considerable concern in Denmark and has led to an array of research projects, including a project by three of us (Andreev, Vaupel, and Yashin) and others at Odense University Medical School. To deepen understanding of Danish mortality relative to mortality in other countries, we are preparing Lexis maps of ratios of mortality in general and of mortality from specific causes, such as cancer or heart disease. Figures 45 and 46 illustrate this line of inquiry. (Lexis maps of mortality and fertility ratios were earlier discussed in section XII of this monograph.)

Figure 45a displays the ratio of age-specific central death rates for males in Denmark vs. Norway, from 1870 through 1993. Figure 45b presents a similar map for females. The red colors indicate higher mortality in Denmark than in Norway; the blue colors indicate lower mortality in Denmark. The darkest red and blue tones denote the ages and times when the discrepencies were greatest. Figures 46a and b are analagous, except they pertain to differences between Denmark and Japan and they cover a much shorter time period--from 1951 through 1991.

Consider, first, the comparison of male mortality in Denmark vs. Norway. Up until and particular during the Second World War, Denmark enjoyed a substantial advantage at ages under 40 or 50. In contrast, Norwegian mortality tended to lower than Danish mortality at older ages up until the mid 1940s, with the striking exception of 1918, the year of the Spanish Influenza epidemic. Over the past half century, both the Danish advantage at younger ages and the Norwegian advantage at older ages have tended to diminish. Between the ages of 30 and 50 there has been a reversal of advantage: between 1920 and 1945 Danish male mortality at these ages was considerably lower than in Norway, but since 1975 it has tended to be considerably higher.

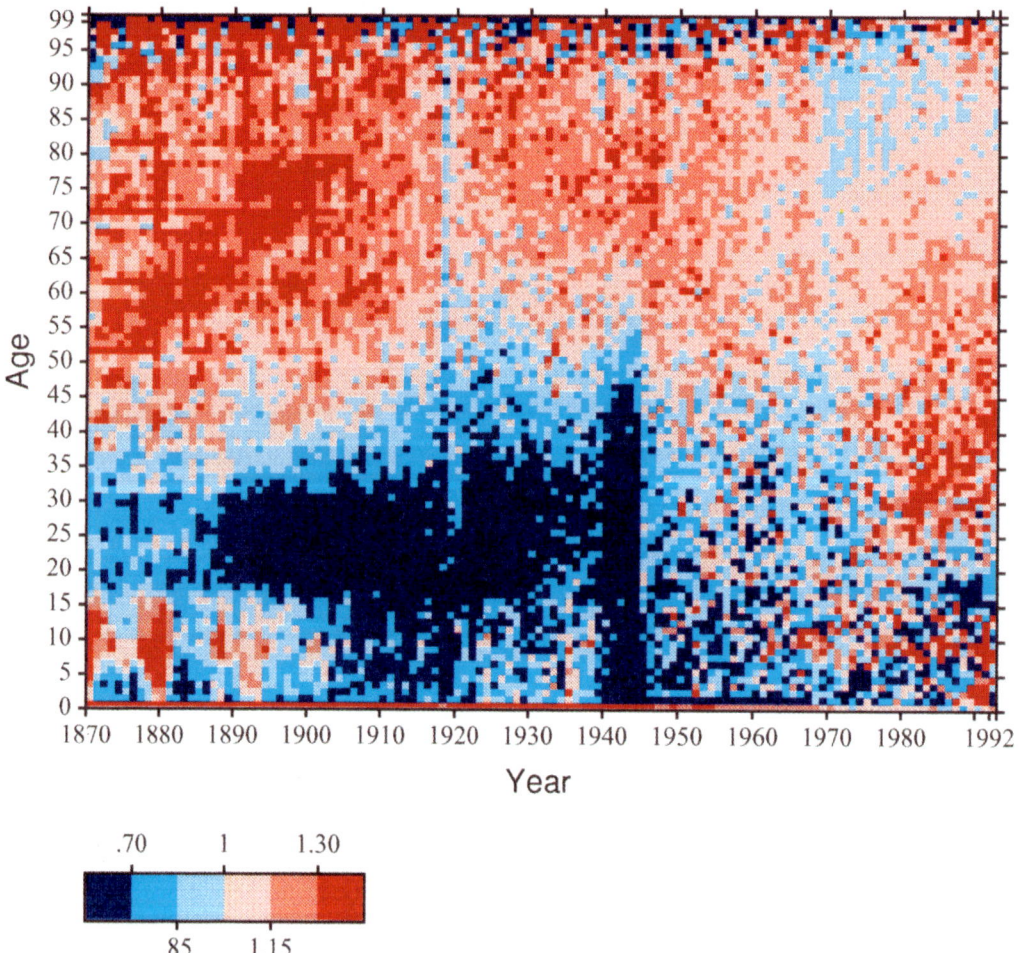

**Figure 45(a).** Ratio of male central death rates in Denmark to those in Norway, with contours selectively placed from 0.7 to 1.3, for age 0 to 99 and year 1870 to 1992.

For females in Denmark vs. Norway the general patterns are roughly similar to the male patterns but with bigger, more striking changes. Note, in particular, the large area of relatively high Danish mortality among middle-aged women that emerges after the Second World War: by 1993 at most ages between 35 and 75 Danish female death rates were more than 30% higher than Norwegian rates. At least some of this domain of disadvantage appears to follow particular birth cohorts. Consider, for instance, the women born in 1930 and age 63 in 1993. This cohort suffered relatively high mortality in almost every year from the mid 1950s.

The map comparing Danish and Japanese males, Figure 46a, also contains some suggestive diagonal blotches of red. The cohorts born around 1960, for instance, who were in their late 20s or early 30s in 1991, had much higher mortality in Denmark than in Japan from age 20 on. Further analysis is needed to determine how much of the

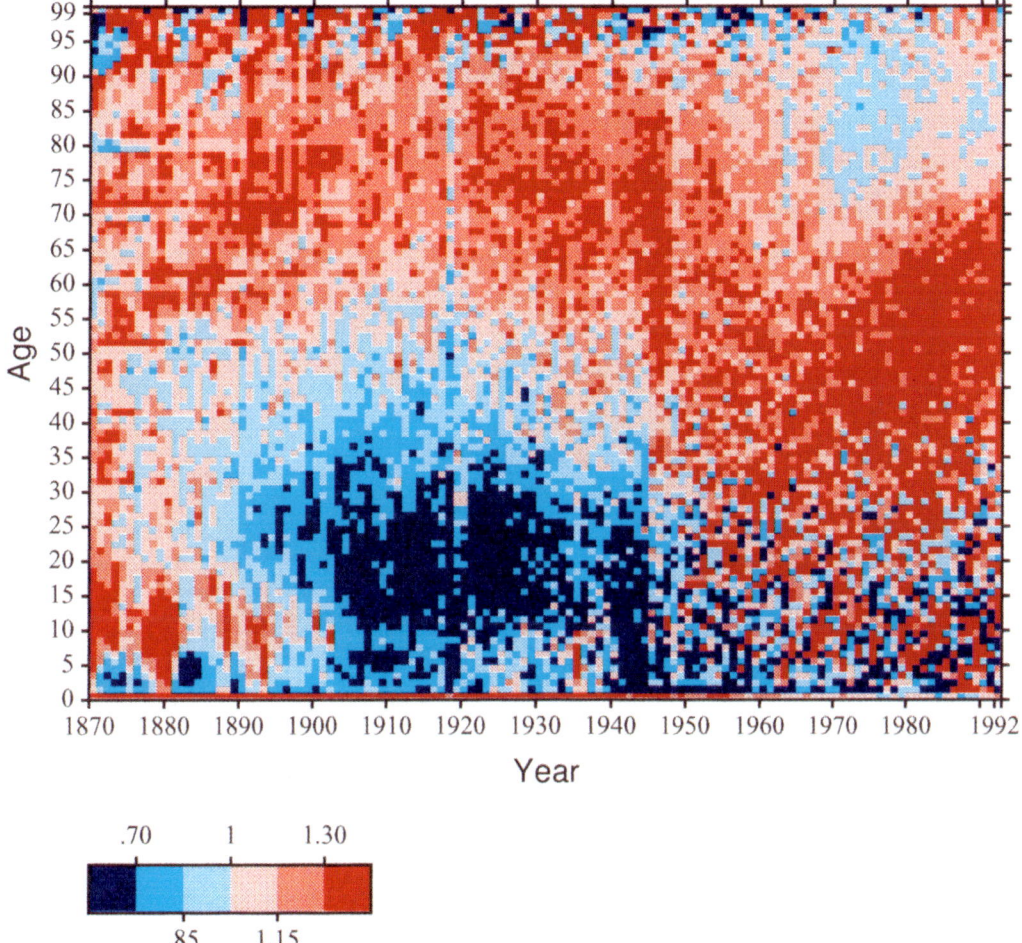

**Figure 45(b).** Ratio of female central death rates in Denmark to those in Norway, with contours selectively placed from 0.7 to 1.3, for age 0 to 99 and year 1870 to 1992.

explanation lies in Danish vs. Japanese mortality trends. Figure 46b, which compares Danish and Japanese female mortality, also contains some hints of cohort patterns. The growing domain of severe Danish disadvantage, starting around age 50 around 1970 and expanding to ages 30 to 80, could also be interpreted as an epidemic-like pattern resulting from the spread of Danish negatives (or, perhaps, Japanese positives) to adjacent age classes.

Viewed in their entirety, the Danish-Japanese comparisons are mostly blue before the early 1970s and mostly red thereafter. The very substantial Danish mortality advantage in earlier years turns into a very substantial Danish mortality disadvantage in more recent years. Japan not only caught up with Denmark but went on to do significantly better than Denmark for both sexes and at almost all ages.

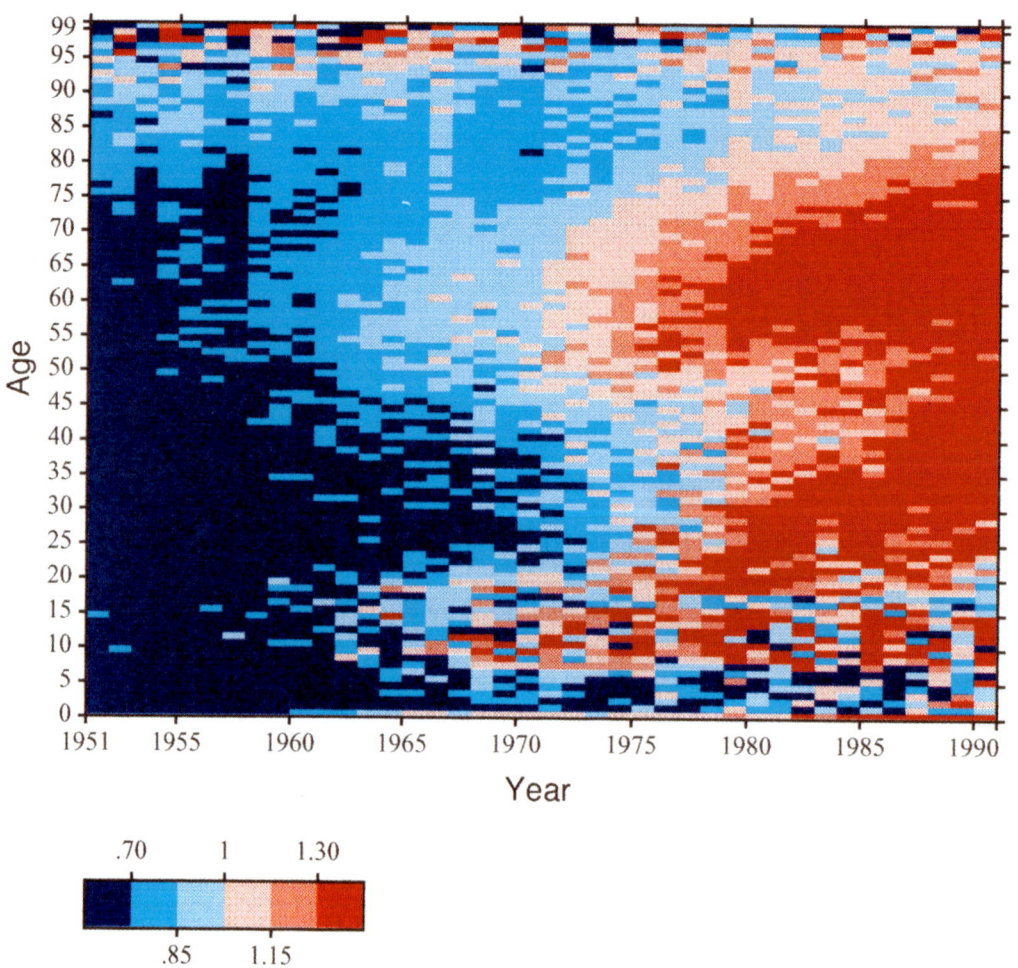

**Figure 46(a).** Ratio of male central death rates in Denmark to those in Japan, with contours selectively placed from 0.7 to 1.3, for age 0 to 99 and year 1951 to 1990.

Further analysis of other mortality comparisons--of Denmark with other countries and Japan with other countries--as well as comparisons of cause-specific mortality could shed new light on how Denmark might reduce death rates. The Lexis maps in Figures 45 and 46 are not only dramatic graphical presentations: they communicate an enormous amount of information in a thought-provoking way.

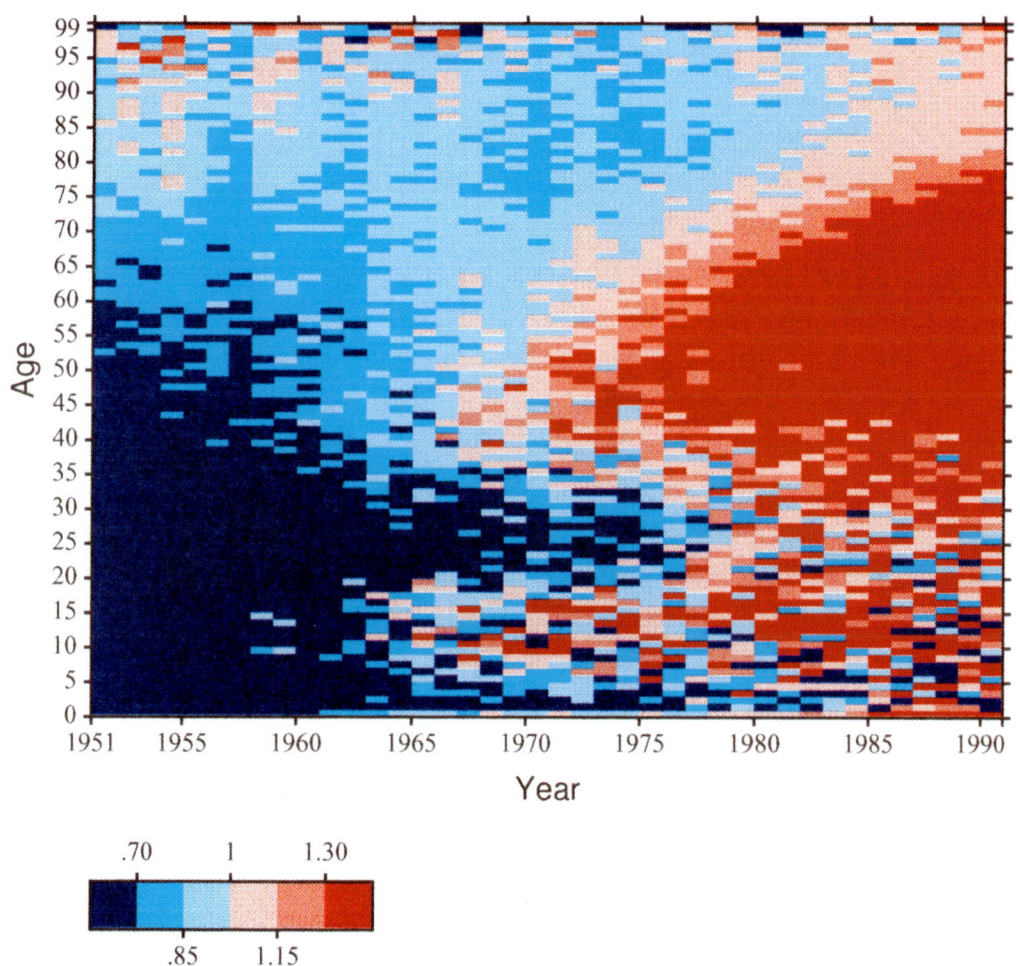

**Figure 46(b).** Ratio of female central death rates in Denmark to those in Japan, with contours selectively placed from 0.7 to 1.3, for age 0 to 99 and year 1951 to 1990.

# 19. Conclusion

The maps presented in this monograph suggest just a few of the numerous ways that demographers can use contour maps to clearly, efficiently, and simultaneously display both persistent global and prominent local patterns in population rates or levels over two dimensions. In particular, contour maps can strikingly reveal the interaction between age, period, and cohort patterns. By using small multiples, computer movies, or ratio surfaces demographers can use the maps to gain access to several dimensions.

Even in cases where some demographic data already have been carefully scrutinized by perceptive analysts who have uncovered most of the interesting patterns, contour maps may be useful in highlighting these patterns. With contour maps, what was before understood now can be seen. Furthermore, the maps, by giving demographers a new perspective on data, may focus attention on some neglected aspects and patterns in even thoroughly studied data.

Beyond efficient description, contour maps can help demographers with exploratory data analysis and with model building. Surfaces can be computed relative to some part of the surface or to another surface; and different surfaces can be placed next to each other and compared. The patterns produced by a model can be displayed for different parameter values as can the fit of the model to some empirical data. If the data are defined over two dimensions, then a contour map can be used to display the residuals, i.e., the differences between the actual values and the values predicted by the model. By scrutinizing the pattern of the residuals, an analyst may glean some clues as to how to improve the model. Tukey (1977) and Mosteller and Tukey (1977) provide clear discussions of the use of residuals in data analysis and model building and several statistical software packages enable users to conveniently plot contour maps of residents.

The resulting contour maps can be displayed not only as printed output but also on a computer monitor. The shades used in most of the maps presented in this monograph range from black to light grey, but the maps can be produced in glowing colors, on a color computer monitor or using a color printer, as illustrated by the 12 color maps included in this monograph and by the maps on the diskette included with the monograph: the effects are dramatic.

Tufte, in his lucid exposition of The Visual Display of Quantitative Information (1983), concludes that graphic designs should give "visual access to the subtle and difficult, that is, the revelation of the complex." Demographic surfaces can be particularly complex. A mortality surface, for example, might be defined over a century of age and a century of time, comprising 10,000 data points that may vary over four orders of magnitude. Contour maps are a striking, efficient, and clear means of giving demographers visual access to such surfaces.

William Playfair (1801), the pioneer of graphical methods for presenting statistical data, argued that with a good visual display "as much information may be obtained in five minutes as would require whole days to imprint on the memory, in a lasting manner, by a table of figures." The 100 Lexis maps in this monograph summarize more than half a million data points in a memorable, revealing manner.

# References

Arthur, W.B., and J.W. Vaupel (1984), Some General Relationships in Population Dynamics, *Population Index* 50(2):214-226.

Bennett, N.G., and S. Horiuchi (1981), Estimating the Completeness of Death Registration in a Closed Population, *Population Index* 47(2):207-221.

Brass, W. (1971), On the Scale of Mortality, in W. Brass (ed.), Biological Aspects of Demography, Taylor and Francis Ltd., London.

Caselli, G., J.W. Vaupel, and A.I. Yashin (1985), Mortality in Italy: Contours of a Century of Evolution, *Genus* 39:1-12.

Caselli, G., J. Vallin, J.W. Vaupel, and A.I. Yashin (1987), Age-Specific Mortality Trends in France and Italy since 1900, *European Journal of Population* 3:20-27.

Coale, A.J., and E.E. Kisker (1985), Mortality Crossovers: Reality or Bad Data?, paper presented at the annual meeting of the Population Association of America, Boston.

Coale, A.J., and E.E. Kister (1990), Defects in Data on Old Age Mortality in the United States, *Asian and Pacific Population Forum* 4(1).

Delaporte, P. (1941), Evolution de la mortalité en Europe depuis l'origine des statistiques de l'Etat civil (Tables de mortalité de générations), Imprimerie Nationale, Paris.

Ewbank, D.C., J.C. Gomez de Leon, and M.A. Stoto (1983), A Reducible Four-Parameter System of Model Life Tables, *Population Studies* 37(1):105-127.

Faber, J.F. (1982), Life Tables for the United States: 1900-2050, Actuarial Study No. 87, U.S. Department of Health and Human Services, SSA Pub. No. 11-11534.

Federici, N. (1955), Lezioni di Demografia, 1 Edizione, De Santis, Roma.

Fisher, H.T. (1982), Mapping Information: The Graphic Display of Quantitative Information, Abt Books, Cambridge, Massachusetts.

Heligman, L., and J.H. Pollard (1980), The Age Pattern of Mortality, *Journal of the Institute of Actuaries* 107(I):49-80.

Heuser, R.L. (1976), Fertility Tables for Birth Cohorts by Color, United States, 1917-1973, U.S. Department of Health Education, and Welfare, National Center for Health Statistics.

Heuser, R.L. (1984), Fertility Tables for Birth Cohorts by Color, United States, 1917-1980, U.S. Department of Health Education, and Welfare, National Center for Health Statistics.

Kannisto, V. (1994), Development of Oldest-Old Mortality, 1950-1990, Odense University Press, Odense, Denmark.

Kannisto, V. (1996), The Advancing Frontier of Survival, Odense University Press, Odense, Denmark.

Kannisto, V., J. Lauritsen, A.R. Thatcher, and J.W. Vaupel (1994), Reductions in Mortality at Advanced Ages, *Population and Development Review* 20(4):793-810.

Kermack, W., A. McKendrick, and P. McKinlay (1934), Death-Rates in Great Britain and Sweden: Some General Regularities and their Significance, *The Lancet* 286:698-703.

Keyfitz, N. (1977), Applied Mathematical Demography, John Wiley & Sons, New York.

Keyfitz, N., and W. Flieger (1968), World Population: An Analysis of Vital Data, University of Chicago Press, Chicago.

Lotka, A.J. (1926), The Progressive Adjustment of Age Distribution to Fecundity, *Journal of the Washington Academy of Sciences* 16(19):505-513.

Lotka, A.J. (1931), The Structure of a Growing Population, *Human Biology* 3(4):459-93.

Mosteller, F., and J.W. Tukey (1977), Data Analysis and Regression: A Second Course in Statistics, Addison-Wesley Co., Reading, Massachusetts.

Natale, M., and A. Bernassola (1973), La mortalita per causa nelle regioni italiane, Tavole per contemporanei 1965-66 e per generazioni 1790-1969, Istituto di Demografia, Universita di Roma, n. 25, Roma.

Perozzo, L. (1880), Della Rappresentazione Grafica di una Collettivita di Individui nella Successione del Tempo, e in Particolare dei Diagrammi a Tre Coordinate, Annali di Statistica Series 2a, Volume 12, Ministry of Agriculture, Industry and Commerce, Rome, Italy.

Playfair, W. (1979), The Commercial and Political Atlas, 3rd ed, p. xii, J. Wallis, London (1801). Quoted in Schmid, C.A. and Schmid, S.E., Handbook of Graphic Presentation, 2nd ed, New York.

Preston, S.H., N. Keyfitz, and R. Schoen (1972), Causes of Death: Life Tables for National Populations, Seminar Press, New York.

Preston, S.H., and E. van de Walle (1978), Urban French Mortality in the Nineteenth Century, *Population Studies* 32(2):275-297.

Preston, S.H., and A.J. Coale (1982), Age Structure, Growth, Attrition, and Accession: A New Synthesis, *Population Index* 48(2):217-259.

Scherbov, S., A.I. Yashin, and V. Grechucha (1986), Dialog System for Modelling Multidimensional Demographic Processes, Working Paper WP-86-29, International Institute for Applied Systems Analysis, Laxenburg, Austria.

Statistics Sweden (1881-1981), Swedish Statistical Yearbooks, Stockholm, Sweden.

Tufte, E.R. (1983), The Visual Display of Quantitative Information, Graphica Press, Cheshire, Connecticut.

Tukey, J.W. (1977), Exploratory Data Analysis, Addison-Wesley Co., Reading Massachusetts.

Vallin, J. (1973), La mortalité par génération en France, depuis 1899, Travaux et Documents, Cahier n. 63, Press Universitaires de France, Paris.

Vaupel, J.W., K. Manton, and E. Stallard (1979), The Impact of Heterogeneity in Frailty on the Dynamics of Mortality, *Demography* 16(3):439-54.

Vaupel, J.W., and H. Lundström (1994), The Future of Mortality at Older Ages in Developed Countries, in W. Lutz (ed.), The Future Population of the World, Eartsean Publications, London.

Vaupel, J.W., and B. Jeune (1995), The Emergence and Proliferation of Centenarians, in B. Jeune (ed.), Exceptional Longevity, Odense University Press, Odense, Denmark.

Veys, D. (1983), Cohort Survival in Belgium in the Past 150 Years, Catholic University of Leuven, Sociological Research Institute, Leuven, Belgium.

Wilmoth, J. (1985), Identifiable Age, Period, and Cohort Effects: An Exploratory Approach Applied to Italian Female Mortality, Working Paper WP-85-69, International Institute for Applied Systems Analysis, Laxenburg, Austria.

Wunsch, G.J., and M.G. Termote (1978), Introduction to Demographic Analysis: Principles and Methods, Plenum Press, New York and London.

Zaba, B. (1979), The Four-Parameter Logit Life-Table System, *Population Studies* 33(1):79-100.

Zeng Y., J.W. Vaupel, and A.I. Yashin (1985), Marriage and Fertility in China: a graphical analysis, *Population and Development Review* 11:721-736.

Zeng Y., J.W. Vaupel, and W. Zhenglian (1995), Marriage and Fertility in China: Graphical Analysis of Recent Trends, *Genus* 49:17-26.